Introduction to Process Evaluation in Tobacco Use Prevention and Control

February 2008

Suggested Citation

Centers for Disease Control and Prevention. *Introduction to Process Evaluation in Tobacco Use Prevention and Control*. Atlanta, GA: U.S. Department of Health and Human Services, Centers for Disease Control and Prevention, National Center for Chronic Disease Prevention and Health Promotion, Office on Smoking and Health; 2008. Available at: http://www.cdc.gov/tobacco/publications/index.htm.

ACKNOWLEDGEMENTS

The manual was prepared by the Centers for Disease Control and Prevention, Office on Smoking and Health.

    Matthew McKenna, Director
    Corinne Husten, Branch Chief, Epidemiology Branch
    Robert Merritt, Team Lead, Evaluation Team

    Donald Compton, Project Lead
    Nicole Kuiper
    Sheila Porter

Contributing Authors

Paul Mattessich, Wilder Research Center
Patricia Rieker, Boston University

Battelle Centers for Public Health Research and Evaluation
    Pamela Clark
    Mary Kay Dugan, Task Leader
    Carol Schmitt

RTI International
    Barri Burrus
    Suzanne Dolina
    Erika Fulmer, Task Leader
    Maria Girlando
    Michelle Myers

We thank the members of the Editorial Review Group and the Expert Panel for contributing their expertise and experience in developing and reviewing this manual.

Editorial Review Group

Centers for Disease Control and Prevention
    Deborah Borbely
    Robert Merritt
    Michael Schooley
    Gabrielle Starr
    Debra Torres

Tobacco Technical Assistance Consortium
    Pamela Redmon

State Health Department Representatives
    Jennifer Ellsworth, Minnesota
    Lois Keithly, Massachusetts
    Mike Placona, North Carolina
    Scott Proescholdbell, North Carolina

Saint Louis University
    Douglas Luke
    Nancy Mueller

Expert Panel

Centers for Disease Control and Prevention

Deborah Borbely
Robert Robinson
Michael Schooley
Brick Lancaster
Patty McLean
Lisa Petersen
Gabrielle Star
Deborah Torres

Michael Baizerman, University of Minnesota
Ursula Bauer, New York Department of Health
Robert Goodman, University of Pittsburgh
Donna Grande, American Medical Association
Paul Mattessich, Wilder Research Center
Edmund Ricci, University of Pittsburgh
Todd Rogers, Public Health Institute
Stacy Scheel, More Voices, Inc.
Laura Linnan, University of North Carolina
Douglas Luke, Saint Louis University
Karla Sneegas, Indiana Tobacco Prevention and Cessation Agency
Frances Stillman, Johns Hopkins University

CDC acknowledges the following National Tobacco Control Program (NTCP) program managers and their staff for participating in interviews to identify key factors associated with successful tobacco use prevention and control programs. We also thank the Ohio Tobacco Use Prevention and Control Foundation for their participation.

Joann Wellman Benson, California
Karen DeLeeuw, Colorado
Joan Stine, Maryland
Lois Keithly, Massachusetts
Paul Martinez, Minnesota
Sally Malek, North Carolina
Terry Reid, Washington
Joan Stine, Ohio
Ken Slenkovitch, Ohio Tobacco Use Prevention and Control Foundation

Contents

Section	Page
Acknowledgements	i
1. Introduction	**1**
1.1 The Planning/Program Evaluation/Program Improvement Cycle	2
1.2 Distinguishing Process Evaluation from Outcome Evaluation	3
2. Purposes and Benefits of Process Evaluation	**4**
2.1 Definition of Process Evaluation	4
2.2 Scope of Tobacco Control Activities Included in a Process Evaluation	4
2.3 Purposes: How Does Process Evaluation Serve You?	4
2.3.1 Program Monitoring	5
2.3.2 Program Improvement	5
2.3.3 Building Effective Program Models	7
2.3.4 Accountability	7
2.4 Users and Uses of Process Evaluation Information	11
2.4.1 Users	11
2.4.2 Uses	14
3. Information Elements Central to Process Evaluation	**17**
3.1 Indicators of Inputs/Activities/Outputs	17
3.2 Comparing Process Information to Performance Criteria	21
4. Managing Process Evaluation	**29**
4.1 Managing Process Evaluation: A 10-Step Process	29
4.1.1 Purpose: Why Use the 10-Step Process for Managing Evaluation?	29
4.1.2 Roles of the Advisory Group, Evaluation Facilitator, and Evaluator	30
4.1.3 Stages and Steps of the 10-Step Process	31
4.1.4 Lessons Learned From Implementing the 10-Step Process	35
4.2 The Program Evaluation Standards and Protecting Participants in Evaluation Research	37
4.2.1 The Program Evaluation Standards	37

Contents

		4.2.2 Protecting Participants in Evaluation Research	38
	4.3	Choosing a Process Evaluation Design (Methodology)	39
	4.4	Process Evaluation—Beyond a Single Study	41

5. Conclusion 43

Glossary of Terms 45

Appendices

A	CDC's Framework for Program Evaluation	47
B	Detailed List of The Joint Committee on Standards for Evaluation: The Program Evaluation Standards	49
C	Additional Information on the Purpose, Selection, and Roles of the Evaluation Advisory Group	53
D	Process Evaluation Questions and Logic Model from the Center for Tobacco Policy Research	57

References 59

EXHIBITS

Number		Page
1-1	CDC's Framework for Program Evaluation	2
1-2	Logic Models	3
2-1	Four Primary Purposes of Process Evaluation	8
3-1	Information Commonly Obtained in a Process Evaluation	18
3-2	Inputs—Comparing Indicators to Criteria	22
3-3	Activities and Outputs—Comparing Indicators to Criteria	24
3-4	Tobacco-Related Disparities: Activities and Outputs—Comparing Indicators to Criteria	25
4-1	Overview of the 10-Step Process for Managing Evaluation	32
4-2	Steps and Staff Responsibilities in the 10-Step Process	33
D-1	Strategy 1 Logic Model: Show Me Health—Clearing the Air About Tobacco	58

Case Examples Based on Logic Model Categories

	Page
Assessment of Learning from truth[sm]: Youth Participation in Field Marketing Techniques to Counter Tobacco Advertising	9
Outcome and Process Evaluation of a School-Based, Informal, Adolescent Peer-Led Intervention to Reduce Smoking	10
Stakeholder Advisory Board: The North Carolina Youth Empowerment Study	13
Assessing the Effectiveness of a Training Curriculum for *Promotores,* Spanish-Speaking Community Health Outreach Workers	14
Assessment of Use of Best Practices Guidelines by 10 State Tobacco Control Programs	15
Incorporating Process Evaluation Findings into Development of a Web-Based Smoking Cessation Program for College-Aged Smokers	16

Case Examples Based on Process Information Components

	Page
Implementation of the Henry J. Kaiser Family Foundation's Community Health Promotion Grant Program	26
New York Statewide School Tobacco Policy Review	27
Elimination of Secondhand Smoke through the Seattle and King County Smoke-Free Housing Initiative	28

1. INTRODUCTION

Tobacco use in the United States is the single most preventable cause of death and disease.[1] The Centers for Disease Control and Prevention's Office on Smoking and Health (CDC/OSH) created the National Tobacco Control Program (NTCP) to foster and support coordinated, nationwide, state-based activities to advance its mission to reduce disease, disability, and death related to tobacco use.

CDC/OSH has identified four program goal areas:

- Preventing initiation of tobacco use among young people;
- Eliminating nonsmokers' exposure to secondhand smoke;
- Promoting quitting among adults and young people; and
- Identifying and eliminating tobacco-related disparities.

To determine the effectiveness of NTCP programs, both their implementation and their outcomes must be measured.[2]

This manual is intended to provide process evaluation technical assistance to OSH staff, grantees and partners. It defines process evaluation and describes the rationale, benefits, key data collection components, and program evaluation management procedures. It also discusses how process evaluation links with outcome evaluation and fits within an overall approach to evaluating comprehensive tobacco control programs. Previous CDC initiatives have provided resources for designing outcome evaluations. (See, for example, the CDC framework depicted in Exhibit 1-1.) This manual complements CDC's approach to outcome evaluation by focusing on process evaluation as a way to document and measure implementation of NTCP programs.

The content of this manual reflects the priorities of CDC/OSH for program monitoring and evaluation, and augments two other CDC/OSH publications: *Key Outcome Indicators for Evaluating Comprehensive Tobacco Control Programs*[3] and *Introduction to Program Evaluation for Comprehensive Tobacco Control Programs.*[2]

This manual:

- Provides a framework for understanding the links between inputs, activities, and outputs and for assessing how these relate to outcomes; and
- Can assist state and federal program managers and evaluation staff with the design and implementation of process evaluations that will provide valid, reliable evidence of progress achieved through their tobacco control efforts.

As you read this manual, keep in mind that it is not a "cookbook" for process evaluation. State and local programs have unique features and contexts that create a need for different types of process-related information. This manual does explain general principles of process evaluation and provides a guide for determining what types of information to gather. Also, be mindful that process evaluation of an overall comprehensive state program such as tobacco control is not typically conducted because the scope of such an evaluation would not be practical and would be extremely costly. Rather, process evaluation is typically used to evaluate a given component or activity within an overall comprehensive program. Finally, please note that for the purposes of this manual, the terms program, project, and intervention are used interchangeably.

1.1 The Planning/Program Evaluation/Program Improvement Cycle

Evaluation is a systematic process to understand what a program does and how well the program does it. Evaluation results can be used to maintain or improve program quality and to ensure that future planning can be more evidence-based. Evaluation constitutes part of an ongoing cycle of program planning, implementation, and improvement.

Exhibit 1-1 provides a visual representation of the six-step CDC framework for general program evaluation.[4] The six steps in the CDC framework represent an ongoing cycle, rather than a linear sequence, and addressing each of the steps is an iterative process.[4] Implicit in the framework is the connection between evaluation and planning. Additional information about each step is provided in Appendix A.

Exhibit 1-1: CDC's Framework for Program Evaluation

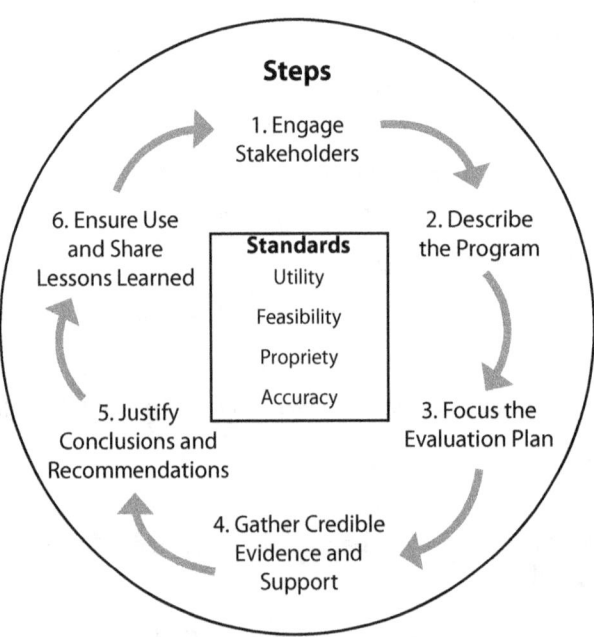

SOURCE: Centers for Disease Control and Prevention. Framework for program evaluation in public health. *MMWR* 1999;48(RR11):1–40.

1.2 Distinguishing Process Evaluation from Outcome Evaluation

The NTCP is guided by logic models which address each of the four goals described earlier. The CDC/OSH approach to tobacco control evaluation is also based in the use of logic models. As shown in **Exhibit 1-2,** logic models specify program inputs, activities, outputs, and outcomes (short-term, intermediate, and long-term).[2,3] (See Glossary for definition of terms.)

Exhibit 1-2: **Logic Models**

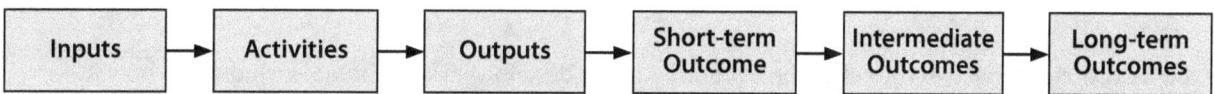

To date, CDC/OSH has developed an approach that emphasizes the last three boxes in **Exhibit 1-2**, focusing on outcomes and providing resources to enable program staff to measure and report them. This is outcome evaluation.

The NTCP has focused on outcome evaluations for several good reasons. Outcome evaluation allows researchers to document health and behavioral outcomes and identify linkages between an intervention and quantifiable effects. Also, epidemiologists and other practitioners often have a well-developed evidence base for population-level intervention outcomes, making it feasible to conduct outcome evaluations.

On the other hand, process evaluation focuses on the first three boxes of the logic model. It enables you to describe and assess your program's activities and to link your progress to outcomes. This is important because the link between outputs and short-term outcomes remains an empirical question. Unlike outcome evaluations, process evaluations often use practice wisdom (that is, the observations and opinions of professionals in the field) to help identify the links between inputs/activities/outputs and short-term outcomes.

A variety of evidence-based guidance is available for NTCP grantees. For example, anticipating the new funds available to states from the 1998 Master Settlement Agreement (MSA), in 1999, CDC/OSH published *Best Practices for Comprehensive Tobacco Control Programs (Best Practices)*.[1] This was the first document to describe the nine core components of a comprehensive tobacco control program. *Best Practices* also contained a formalized set of funding recommendations which helped shape state tobacco control programs by providing national frameworks and standards.[5] Since *Best Practices* was released, new guides and reviews have been published. For instance, the *Guide to Community Preventive Services*,[6] and the *California Communities of Excellence in Tobacco Control*[7] establish planning frameworks that help to define state activities, expected outputs, and standards useful for process evaluation. We have included an example of an actual logic model for a process evaluation (Appendix D), which was provided by the Center for Tobacco Policy Research (CTPR), Saint Louis University School of Public Health.

2. PURPOSES AND BENEFITS OF PROCESS EVALUATION

This chapter is intended to answer fundamental questions about the value and implementation of process evaluation within tobacco use prevention and control efforts.

2.1 Definition of Process Evaluation

Process evaluation, as one aspect of overall program evaluation, is:

> The systematic collection of information on a program's inputs, activities, and outputs, as well as the program's context and other key characteristics.

Process evaluation involves the collection of information to describe what a program includes and how it functions over time. In and of itself, the information is "neutral." It is merely descriptive, although people often attach meaning and value to the information. It does not reflect "quality" until you compare it to an external set of standards or criteria.

Process evaluations can occur just once, periodically throughout the duration of a program, or continuously. The type of information gathered, and its frequency, will depend on the kinds of questions that you seek to answer.

2.2 Scope of Tobacco Control Activities Included in a Process Evaluation

In evaluations of tobacco-control programs, a question commonly arises: On what "level of program(s) or activities" should the evaluation focus? The answer is: The number and type of programs and activities included in a process evaluation will depend on the interests and questions of stakeholders and the intended uses of the information.

For example, if the objective of a process evaluation is solely to assess the efforts of a particular program (e.g., efforts to increase the cigarette tax or increase use of a quitline), and to improve that program, then a process evaluation will gather information related only to that program. On the other hand, if the purpose of a process evaluation is to assess comprehensive tobacco control efforts within a community, a state, or some other geographic region, then a process evaluation will gather information related to all of the varied programs in the specified geographic area. As another example, a number of states have already passed smoke-free work place laws; thus the objective of a process evaluation might be to assess the education, training, and technical assistance provided to interpret and implement these laws.

2.3 Purposes: How Does Process Evaluation Serve You?

Process evaluation has four primary purposes related to individual programs and to the general field of tobacco control: program monitoring, program improvement, development of effective program models, and accountability. This section provides a brief overview of these purposes, along with case examples. Later in this manual, you will find more examples, as well as details on the information you can collect to fulfill these purposes.

2.3.1 Program Monitoring

Program monitoring includes tracking, documenting, and summarizing the inputs, activities, and outputs of your program. So, for example, you may record at one or more points in time:

- How much money is spent,
- The number of staff and/or volunteers involved in the activities of the program,
- The amount and types of activities related to tobacco use prevention and control,
- The number or proportion of people reached,
- The economic, social, and demographic characteristics of people reached, and
- The number of meetings or training sessions conducted.

Second, program monitoring includes the description of characteristics of the program and its context, which might be important for understanding how and why it worked the way it did. For example, you might note:

- The locale where a program carries out its activities (e.g., rural, urban),
- Demographic or economic characteristics of the target population of the program,
- Amount of training that staff received,
- Age of the program at the time of the evaluation, and
- Unique events that occurred during the course of a program's efforts.

Careful, reliable monitoring of the inputs, activities, and outputs of your program—along with a description of the program's characteristics and context—provides the basic, elemental data necessary for process evaluation. Such information enables you to determine what you are doing; you can use this information on its own, and you can use it in connection with the other three purposes of process evaluation or link it with outcomes.

Later, we discuss specific data that process evaluations usually collect for program monitoring. Note, however, that no hard and fast rules apply to the selection of data to collect. The information that you need will depend on the questions you want to answer.

2.3.2 Program Improvement

Once you have information about inputs, activities, and outputs, along with information on the characteristics and context of a program, you can use this information to support decisions regarding program improvement or future planning.

Consider the example of a quitline program. For those individuals who actually make contact and complete the program, it may be achieving good quit rates. However, suppose the program suffers from insufficient recruitment and retention of participants. Process evaluation can reveal why participation levels fall short of program objectives. For instance, results may show that the program has some inconvenient features, lacks optimal language or cultural attributes, or has other characteristics that create barriers. You and your fellow program managers can then use these findings to improve the quitline by increasing participation and completion.

In using process evaluation for program improvement, you will most commonly approach your task in either or both of two ways:

a. Comparing a program to a standard or expectation (e.g., program goals/objectives, funding recommendations and guidelines, or standards of practice).

    You can compare any of the data that you obtain in a process evaluation to the specific goals or objectives of your program. For example, you may have targets regarding the number or type of people you will reach or the amount of service that you will provide. Process evaluation will show whether you are meeting those targets; if not, you can adjust your efforts accordingly.

    Process information (e.g., information on the types of persons reached by the program, languages spoken, features of the program) can help you understand whether you are reaching specific populations. Process information can also support your decision-making regarding the best ways to adapt or fine tune the program to appeal to the broadest array of persons in the intended population.

    "Evidence-based" or "best practice" standards [1,6] sometimes exist for a program. When they do, you can compare your performance to these standards, using process evaluation information. (This is sometimes called assessing "fidelity" to established practice standards.) If you discover a lack of alignment with established standards or guidelines, you can adjust your program for a better fit. In the absence of standards derived from evidence-based research, normative standards can be developed based on the experience of programs of a similar type. For example, if you are planning a print media campaign, you may learn from other programs that multi-media campaigns are more effective than print media alone.

b. Relating process data to outcome data.

    Program outcome data enable you to know whether you are producing the desired effects. You can examine your outcome evaluation data and process evaluation data together to identify steps you can take to increase effectiveness.

    In fact, process evaluation is most effective when implemented in conjunction with outcome evaluation. Knowing what actually occurred as the program was implemented helps you to understand and analyze the conditions that are responsible for a given outcome. Ideally, process evaluation will allow you to attribute strengths and/or weaknesses of your program to specific program characteristics or activities. Without this information, you may find it very difficult to take action when attempting to improve the program using only outcome information.[8]

2.3.3 Building Effective Program Models

The experiences of multiple programs have shown that the tobacco control field can use process and outcome information jointly to build effective program models. Evaluation research can identify, for example, which activities tend to lead to the best outcomes. This use of process evaluation typically lies outside the purview of a single program, unless that program is large enough to vary its activities systematically and test how that variation affects outcomes. More commonly, individual programs will simply report their process and outcome data to CDC/OSH or in annual reports; or they might participate in a controlled or natural field experiment.

Controlled scientific experiments to validate evidence-based practices can incorporate process evaluation for multiple functions. For example, documentation of inputs and activities produces information for comparing the extent to which experimental and control programs have carried out their work in conformity with study protocols. Accurate recording of outputs enables researchers to compare the relative productivity of experimental and control programs. Documentation of activities, as well as unique occurrences that affected a specific program, can assist in the interpretation of experimental data, in the explanation of anomalies, and in decisions concerning validity of specific cases to be included in the analysis of an experiment's findings. See also Steckler and Linnan (2002)[9] for a discussion of process evaluation in the development of theory-based interventions.

2.3.4 Accountability

Process evaluation assists a program in being accountable to its funders, regulators, and other stakeholders, including government officials and policy makers. It does so, first of all, by providing the data necessary to justify expenditures of time and money—for example, demonstrating the number of materials produced, the amount of public advertising, the number of people reached or served, and so forth. A clear demonstration of the links between program inputs, activities, and outcomes enhances justification for funding.

Second, process evaluation supports accountability by documenting compliance with externally imposed standards[1] or criteria established by program funders for continued funding of the program. For example, process evaluation can indicate whether staffing for a program meets the level recommended by CDC.

See **Exhibit 2-1** for more information on the purposes of process evaluation and examples of questions that process evaluation enables you to answer.

---

[1] These standards are often based on research that has established evidence-based practice, but not necessarily.

Exhibit 2-1: Four Primary Purposes of Process Evaluation

Purpose	What You Can Do with Process Evaluation	Sample Questions
1. Program monitoring	Track, document, and summarize the inputs, activities, and outputs of a program. Describe other relevant characteristics of the program and/or its context.	• How much money do we spend on this program? • What activities are taking place? • Who is conducting the activities? • How many people do we reach? • What types of people do we reach? • How much effort (e.g., meetings, media volume, etc.) did we put into a program or specific intervention that we completed?
2. Program improvement	Compare the inputs, activities, and outputs of your program to standards or criteria, your expectations/plans, or recommended practice (fidelity). Relate information on program inputs, activities, and outputs to information on program outcomes.	• Do we have the right mix of activities? • Are we reaching the intended targets? • Are the right people involved as partners, participants, and providers? • Do the staff/volunteers have the necessary skills?
3. Building effective program models	Assess how process is linked to outcomes to identify the most effective program models and components.	• What are the strengths and weaknesses within discrete components of a multi-level program? • What is the optimal path for achieving a specific result (e.g., getting smoke-free regulations passed)?
4. Program accountability	Demonstrate to funders and other decision makers that you are making the best possible use of program resources.	• Have the program inputs or resources been allocated or mobilized efficiently?

In the following case examples, tobacco control professionals have found process evaluation useful for assisting with practical issues they face in implementing high quality programs. (Note that these case examples, as well as the others later in this manual, are tied to specific parts of a logic model and/or to the categories of information typically gathered in a process evaluation. This link to the model is intended to strengthen the use of process evaluation within the overall CDC approach to evaluation.)

CASE EXAMPLE BASED ON LOGIC MODEL CATEGORY: *ACTIVITIES*

Assessment of Learning from truth®: Youth Participation in Field Marketing Techniques to Counter Tobacco Advertising

The **truth®** campaign, a mass-media (print and television) counter-marketing activity targeting youth age 12-17, was funded by the American Legacy Foundation and included a national field marketing component (the **truth®** tour). This unique campaign promotes an "edgy youth" brand and provides information about tobacco, the tobacco industry, and the social costs of tobacco use. It advocates that teens take control of their lives and reject the influence of the industry's advertising practices. The goal is to reach non-mainstream teens, a group that evidence shows to be at risk for smoking initiation, by using youth who reflect the target audience to staff a field marketing endeavor."

How process evaluation was helpful:

The tour was designed to encourage direct youth-to-youth contact to facilitate the transmission of tobacco counter-marketing information. This unique approach posed several problems for a traditional outcome evaluation design. The age of the target audience precluded follow-up interviews without parental permission, so an ethnographic approach was used to provide process evaluation data instead. Methods consisted of observation, participant-observation, informal conversations, and semistructured and unstructured open-ended interviews with the tour riders, staff, and adults from the visited communities.

The purpose of the evaluation was program improvement. Data were needed to document tour activities and group dynamics, and to assess the impact of tour participation on the riders. Riders consisted of three groups of between 6 and 12 carefully selected, diverse, and specially trained youth (under the age of 18) who visited 27 cities in 2000. The tour created three small, close-knit mobile communities who lived and worked together for a 6-week period. The tour was built around high visibility trucks painted with the **truth®** logo and specific music geared to appeal to the targeted audience in selected venues. To avoid undermining the edgy youth image, no one from the local markets was involved in the planning or implementation of tour activities.

Advantages for you:

The evaluation provided an opportunity to assess the implementation of a unique field marketing approach to reaching teens with a public health message about tobacco use. Evaluation results highlight various lessons learned. The evaluation provided an in-depth understanding of the range and type of difficulties associated with underage, "edgy" culturally diverse riders. A possible alternative would be to hire young adults who do not need to be supervised as closely while on the road and to involve youth from local markets in the planning and implementation of the activity. The latter would address the problems that occurred with visiting venues where none of the target audience appeared. Sensitivity training around issues of race, ethnicity, sexual preference, and youth culture is required for all adult staff when traveling on the road with diverse youth. Evaluation results also suggest that field marketing techniques for a national social marketing campaign can benefit from involvement of a local distribution system for the product or message, in order to create linkages that might sustain brand visibility and product availability in the community. Closer ties with local level tobacco control allies who reflect the image of the campaign would be a more effective strategy.

SOURCE: Eisenberg M, Ringwalt C, Driscoll D, Vallee M, Gullette G. Learning from truth®: Youth participation in field marketing techniques to counter tobacco advertising. Journal of Health Communication 2004; 9:223-231.

(Continued)

CASE EXAMPLE BASED ON LOGIC MODEL CATEGORY: *ACTIVITIES and OUTPUTS*

Outcome and Process Evaluation of a School-Based, Informal, Adolescent Peer-Led Intervention to Reduce Smoking

Peer education as a strategy for youth health promotion is used extensively, although there is mixed evidence for its effectiveness. There are few systematic accounts of what young people actually do as peer educators. To examine the activities of the young people recruited as "peer supporters" for A Stop Smoking in Schools Trial (ASSIST) in southeast Wales and the West of England, 10,730 students in 59 secondary schools were recruited at baseline. The ASSIST peer nomination procedure was successful in recruiting, training, and retaining influential year 8 peer supporters of both genders to intervene informally to reduce smoking levels in their year group.

How process evaluation was helpful:

Outcome data at 1-year follow-up showed that the risk of students who were occasional or experimental smokers at baseline reporting weekly smoking at follow-up was 18.2% lower in the intervention schools. This result was supported by analysis of salivary cotinine. To understand how this short-term outcome was achieved, researchers assessed qualitative data from the process evaluation. These data showed that the majority of peer supporters adopted a pragmatic strategy: they concentrated their attention on friends and peers who were occasional or non-smokers and whom they felt could be persuaded not to take up smoking regularly, rather than those they considered to be already "addicted" or who were members of smoking cliques.

Advantages for you:

By combining process and outcome evaluation, the authors were able to identify how the peer supporters actually implemented the intervention to achieve the outcome. The study showed that school-based peer educators are effective in diffusing health promotion messages when they are asked to work informally rather than under the structured supervision of teaching staff. The smoking behavior of the peer supporters themselves also appears to have been affected by the training. Though not encouraged to use fear-based approaches (as best practice would suggest) the peer educators actually employed such tactics effectively. While the message delivered by the peer educators was relatively unsophisticated and soon appeared to lose momentum, a two-year follow-up will substantiate whether the reduction in smoking levels is maintained.

SOURCE: Audrey A, Holliday J, Campbell R. It's good to talk: Adolescent perspectives of an informal, peer-led intervention to reduce smoking. *Social Science and Medicine* 2006;63:320-334.

2.4 Users and Uses of Process Evaluation Information

2.4.1 Users

There are three major groups of stakeholders integral to program evaluation:

- Those served or affected by the program, such as patients or clients, advocacy groups, community members, and elected officials;

- Those involved in program operations, such as management, program staff, partners, the funding agency or agencies, and coalition members; and

- Those in a position to make decisions about the program, such as partners, the funding agency, coalition members, and the general public.

A primary feature of an effective evaluation is the identification of the intended users who can most directly benefit from an evaluation.[8] A first step should be to identify evaluation stakeholders, including those who have a stake or vested interest in evaluation results, as well as those who have a direct or indirect interest in program effectiveness.[8] Identification and engagement of intended users in the evaluation process will help increase use of evaluation information. These intended users are more likely to understand and feel ownership in the evaluation process if they have been actively involved in it.[8] Additionally, such engagement enhances understanding and acceptance of the utility of evaluation information throughout the lifecycle of a program. So, to ensure that information collected, analyzed, and reported successfully meets the needs of stakeholders, you should work with the people who will be using this information from the beginning of the evaluation process and focus on how they will use it to answer what kind of questions.

The following are possible stakeholders in tobacco prevention and control programs:

- Program managers and staff

- Local, state, and regional coalitions interested in reducing tobacco use

- Local recipients of tobacco-related funds

- Local and national partners (such as the American Cancer Society, the American Lung Association, the American Heart Association, the Centers for Disease Control and Prevention, the American Legacy Foundation, the Substance Abuse and Mental Health Services Administration, and the Robert Wood Johnson Foundation)

- Funding agencies, such as national and state governments or foundations

- State or local health departments and health commissioners

- State education agencies, schools, and educational groups

- Universities and educational institutions

- Local government, state legislators, and state governors

- Privately owned businesses and business associations
- Health care systems and the medical community
- Religious organizations
- Community organizations
- Private citizens
- Program critics
- Representatives of populations disproportionately affected by tobacco use
- Law enforcement representatives

As you review this list, consider that many of these stakeholders have diverse and, at times, competing interests. Given that a single evaluation cannot answer all possible issues raised by these diverse interests, the list of stakeholders must be narrowed to a more specific group of primary intended evaluation users; the recommended number of primary intended evaluation users is 8-10.[10] These stakeholders/primary intended users will serve in advisory roles on all phases of the evaluation, beginning with identification of primary intended uses of the evaluation (see Section 4).

To identify the primary intended users, you and your program collaborators should identify all possible stakeholders and determine how critical it is for the findings of the evaluation to influence each stakeholder. Only those stakeholders whom you want to be influenced and to take action (as opposed to those for whom information is valuable to know, but not critical) should be included as primary intended users.

CASE EXAMPLE BASED ON LOGIC MODEL CATEGORY: *INPUTS*

Stakeholder Advisory Board
The North Carolina Youth Empowerment Study

The North Carolina Youth Empowerment Study (NC YES) was a three-year participatory evaluation of youth-based tobacco use prevention programs. The study aimed to document the characteristics of youth tobacco use and prevention programs throughout North Carolina, and to track the role youth in these programs played in implementing tobacco-free policies within local school districts.

How process evaluation was helpful:

One important component of the project involved convening an advisory board of key program stakeholders, including both youth and adults. The purpose of the advisory board was to provide input on all aspects of the study, including the study's research questions, data collection strategies, and interpretation of results. Board members were selected to reflect the racial, ethnic, and geographic diversity of the state, as well as the diversity within types of participating organizations.

Advantages for you:

The benefits of this collaboration were apparent to both researchers and stakeholders who were members of the advisory board. For example, the research team was able to use the board's input on the data collection tools so that the information collected would be of greater use to the community. The board also requested that the research team disseminate results beyond the university so that a wider audience would have access to the findings. Being involved in the process benefited board members through increased knowledge of evaluation and research methods. They also felt that their experiences and skills had been utilized through the participatory process and that the information disseminated benefited multiple audiences, not just the research community.

SOURCE: Ribisl KM, Steckler A, Linnan L, Patterson CC, Pevzner E, Markatos E, et al. The North Carolina Youth Empowerment Study (NC YES): A participatory research study examining the impact of youth empowerment for tobacco use prevention. *Health Education & Behavior* 2004;31(5):597–614.

> **CASE EXAMPLE BASED ON LOGIC MODEL CATEGORY:** *ACTIVITIES*
>
> **Assessing the Effectiveness of a Training Curriculum for *Promotores*, Spanish-Speaking Community Health Outreach Workers**
>
> Tobacco Free El Paso's objective was to recruit and train *promotores* who would deliver comprehensive tobacco cessation interventions (including free nicotine replacement therapies) to low-income, predominantly Spanish-speaking populations of smokers. Although *promotores* are used along the U.S.-Mexico Border to conduct health education classes on topics related to diabetes and other health-related conditions, there is no research on what role they can play as tobacco cessation counselors.
>
> **How process evaluation was helpful:**
>
> The training courses (each of which lasted five days) offered three levels of certification: an introductory basic skills level; intermediate treatment specialist; and, advanced "leave the addiction" specialist. Over a one-year period (August 2003–August 2004), 24 training courses involving 89 participants were delivered. Process information was obtained on the 74 participants who were certified for the introductory level. Of these, 39 went on to the intermediate level and 34 to the advanced certification. To determine the course's effect on self-confidence and satisfaction, participants were given pre- and post-test measures. While self-confidence improved in all participants, those who completed all the three levels showed the most significant increase and were judged capable of delivering a brief smoking cessation intervention. High satisfaction scores indicated that participants felt adequately prepared.
>
> Program staff used this information to validate the program's success and to improve implementation of their "train the trainer" model. The fact that the training courses were easily accessible and free of charge increased attendance. But the length of the course had a deterrent effect as indicated by the smaller number who completed the higher levels of training. As a result, the 5-day training session was shortened to 1-, 2-, and 3-day sessions in order increase the number of participants who advance to the higher training levels. This change was necessary to accommodate participants' diverse work schedules.
>
> **Advantages for you:**
>
> *Promotores* who successfully completed the entire program became part of an extended "train the trainer" team, with the intention of producing broad population change, and reducing disparities for low-income, Spanish-speaking people in El Paso. Program staff used the process information to refine the program's activities and maximize the number of *promotores* who would undergo the full training program. Similarly, you can monitor activities, record participation, and assess satisfaction in order to adjust programs systematically to eliminate problems that might be reducing your effectiveness.
>
> SOURCE: Martinez-Bristow Z, Sias JJ, Urquidi U, Feng C. Tobacco cessation services through community health workers for Spanish-speaking populations. *American Journal of Public Health, Field Action Report* 2006;96(2): 211-213.

2.4.2 Users

As discussed earlier in this chapter, process evaluations can serve a variety of purposes and can be useful in different ways. Below are two examples of how ongoing process evaluations were used to improve program guidance and programmatic activities.

Section 2—Purposes and Benefits of Process Evaluation

CASE EXAMPLE BASED ON LOGIC MODEL CATEGORY: *INPUTS*

Assessment of Use of Best Practices Guidelines by 10 State Tobacco Control Programs

The *Best Practices for Comprehensive Tobacco Control Programs* developed by CDC/OSH in 1999 was the first national resource to define the required components of a comprehensive tobacco control program. The guidelines provide a framework for planning and implementing tobacco control activities. The questions addressed in the qualitative process evaluation were whether and how states used the guidelines in their program planning, and what strengths and weaknesses of the guidelines could be identified. During 2002-2003, process evaluation data were collected and analyzed from 10 state tobacco control programs on familiarity, funding, and use of the guidelines. Information was obtained through written surveys and qualitative interviews with key tobacco partners in the states. The typical number of participants interviewed was 17, representing an average of 15 agencies per state.

How process evaluation was helpful:

The results showed that lead agencies and advisory agencies were most familiar with the guidelines, while other state agencies were less aware of them. Most states modified the guidelines to develop frameworks that were tailored to their context. For example, many states prioritized the nine components and expenditures according to their own available resources because funding levels were not always realistic.

Advantages for you:

The results show that the strength of the guidelines included providing a basic framework for program planning and specific funding recommendations. Limitations included the fact that the guidelines did not address implementation strategies or tobacco-related disparities, and had not been updated with current evidence-based research. To ensure that the guidelines continued to be useful to the states, the evaluators recommended that the guidelines be updated to address implementation of program components, identify strategies to reduce tobacco-use disparities, and include evidence-based examples. Recommended funding levels also need to be revised to be more effective in changing social and political climates, and, the guidelines need to be disseminated beyond typical lead agencies to other tobacco control partners, such as coalitions and relevant state agencies.

SOURCE: Mueller N, Luke D, Herbers S, Montgomery T. The best practices: Use of the guidelines by ten state tobacco control programs. American Journal of Preventive Medicine 2006;31(4).

Introduction to Process Evaluation in Tobacco Use Prevention and Control

---

CASE EXAMPLE BASED ON LOGIC MODEL CATEGORY: *ACTIVITIES*

Incorporating Process Evaluation Findings into Development of a Web-Based Smoking Cessation Program for College-Aged Smokers

College-aged smokers often do not use traditional cessation methods, such as support groups and counseling, to reduce their levels of smoking. Therefore, this study aimed to explore the option of an Internet-based cessation intervention, Kick It!, designed especially for college students. The purpose of the study was to develop the system and conduct a process evaluation to understand usage and acceptability of the intervention, as well as to obtain other feedback.

How process evaluation was helpful:

Thirty-five smokers participated in the intervention, and the research team conducted qualitative interviews with 6 of the 35 students. The interviews were designed to obtain more information on student use of the Kick It! program, their thoughts on the program's strengths and weaknesses, and their recommendations for future change. The in-depth interviews uncovered several useful suggestions for adding components to the program, creating a more personalized system, and making format and content changes.

Advantages for you:

The information collected from respondents was detailed enough to allow Kick It! developers to improve the program for future users and for other researchers to review the work conducted through this process evaluation to inform development of similar programs for college-aged students.

SOURCE: Escoffery C, McCormick L, Bateman K. Development and process evaluation of a Web-based smoking cessation program for college smokers: Innovative tool for education. Patient Education and Counseling 2003; 53:217–5.

3. INFORMATION ELEMENTS CENTRAL TO PROCESS EVALUATION

3.1 Indicators of Inputs/Activities/Outputs

In a process evaluation, you will collect indicators related to the first three categories of an evaluation logic model (inputs, activities, and outputs):[2]

- *Input indicators* measure the various resources that go into a program. Inputs for a tobacco control program can relate to staffing, funds, and other resources.

- *Activity indicators* measure the actual events that take place as part of a program. In tobacco control, these events could include youth education campaigns, messages delivered via the media, coalition development, and many other types of efforts.

- *Output indicators* measure the direct products of a program's activities. Examples include the number of participants using a smoking quitline, a completed media campaign, a higher cigarette tax, the number of posters placed in stores and buses, and other products.

The following table (Exhibit 3-1) lists typical information elements gathered through process evaluation, describes them, and provides examples of measures or indicators[2] that can provide this information. The first three sets of information elements appear within the categories of inputs, activities, and outputs. Next, some additional information elements that relate holistically to the overall program and/or its context are listed.

Note that the types of information you collect will depend on the program's objectives and should be related to the questions the process evaluation will address. For example, it is typically very important to obtain information on the characteristics of persons reached or otherwise affected by your program or policy/regulations. However, which characteristics will you choose to monitor? Gender? Ethnicity? Age? In designing your process evaluation, the characteristics you select to measure will depend on your specific information needs. So, for example, if an evidence-based program applies only to a specific age group, you will want to measure age; or if you need to understand differences in outcomes among persons of different ethnic backgrounds, then you will want to measure ethnicity.

---

[2] In some cases, a single information element constitutes an indicator on its own (e.g., the number of staff). In other cases, two or more elements combine to make a meaningful indicator (e.g., dollars spent per capita).

Exhibit 3-1: Information Commonly Obtained in a Process Evaluation

Item	Description	Example Process Indicators[1]
Inputs		
Financial	Revenues to support prevention and control activities, by source; costs (total or specific to each activity)	Expenses for staff, supplies, media, etc. Dollars spent per capita. Sources of funds
Personnel—Quantity	The number of paid staff and/or volunteers involved; hours of paid staff and volunteers	Number of staff who carry out the prevention/control activities. Hours of effort to produce a product
Personnel—Professional Characteristics	Qualifications/experience/training of staff/volunteers involved	Number of staff with special certification. Educational background of staff and volunteers
Personnel—Personal Characteristics	Individual characteristics of staff/volunteers involved	Ethnic background of staff. Age of staff. Gender of staff
Facilities	Key characteristics of the building(s) and equipment	Hours of operation. Accessibility. Technological capability
Locale	Location where the initiative occurs or the program operates	Geographic scope of prevention/control activities. Neighborhood type (e.g., urban)
Activities		
Population-oriented prevention activity	Description of activities to discourage use or exposure voluntarily, or to eliminate use or exposure legally—focused on the community or a segment of the community	Whether and how counter-marketing occurs. Whether and how information is presented to legislators. Whether and how technical assistance is provided to agencies
Individual-oriented activity	Description of activities directed toward individuals, on an individual basis or in defined groups	Type of training. Type of counseling
Accessibility	Characteristics of the program that facilitate exposure to the intervention	Language of campaign materials. Time of day that program is offered. Languages spoken by staff and/or volunteers. Proximity to mass transit
Recruitment	Processes for identifying, approaching, and engaging targeted audience	Type of contact. Means of advertising. Incentives used to engage audience

Exhibit 3-1: Information Commonly Obtained in a Process Evaluation (continued)

Item	Description	Example Process Indicators
Outputs		
Persons reached	The number of people with documented exposure to messages or who participate in prevention/control activities	Number of people reached Number of class participants
Characteristics of persons reached	Demographic, family, personal, health, and other attributes of the people reached by prevention/control activities	Age Gender Comparison of characteristics of persons reached with characteristics of the intended target population
Products resulting from prevention/control activities	Amount of messages, public meetings, advertisements, promotional segments in TV, radio, newspapers; and, if applicable, service units delivered	Number of advertisements Amount of donated air time Number of meetings with legislators Number of course sessions Number of public meetings Gross Rating Points (GRPs)
Documents that influence tobacco control in a target area	Written plans, guidelines, or other documents that influence the pattern of tobacco control activities (systems, partnerships, campaigns, service delivery) within a target area	Completed state plan
Other Elements Relating to an Initiative/Program as a Whole or to its Context		
Developmental stage	Description of program's maturity/current stage of activities	Stage, e.g.: • Formative/planning • Early implementation • Established but still being modified • Established but stable • In decline
Organizational structure and components	Description of the makeup of the organization, task force, coalition, etc., that oversees and implements program activities, including accountability for distinct activity modules, as well as other relevant structural, leadership, service delivery, and/or administrative processes	• Name(s) of organization(s) involved, overall and for each major portion of the activities • Affiliations of managers • Type of inter-agency agreement, if any

(Continued)

Exhibit 3-1: **Information Commonly Obtained in a Process Evaluation (continued)**

Item	Description	Example Process Indicators
Program theory and fidelity	Presence or absence of elements/characteristics of tobacco prevention/control activities that have been specified through previous research, guidelines, and the development of protocols	• Checklist of steps or guidelines specified in best practice instructions • Chronology of significant implementation actions • Identification of events that interfered with planned activities or implementation of activities
Collaborations/partnerships	Extent to which a program involves multiple independent agencies joined in a formal arrangement and mutually accountable for all or part of the work	• Membership lists • Inter-agency agreements • Roles of each partner • Survival of the collaboration for the duration of the activities
Social, political, economic environment in area of focus for the tobacco prevention/control activities	Elements of the social, political, and economic conditions that affect the planning, implementation, and/or evaluation of the activities intended to be implemented by a program	• Opinions about tobacco control in legislature or among the general public • Major economic trends in area • Legislation/regulations that enhance or impede tobacco prevention/control activities • Tobacco industry activities and promotions
Other unique occurrences	Events within or outside of a program that affect its implementation or ongoing operations	• Disruptive social, historical, or environmental events that influence program activities, accessibility, or reach • Delays in acquisition of financial resources, staff, equipment, etc.

3.2 Comparing Process Information to Performance Criteria

The specific information elements you collect will depend both on the type of tobacco prevention/control activities you intend to implement as well as the questions you need to answer through your process evaluation. As mentioned earlier, process information, in and of itself, is neutral. It does not indicate quality, fidelity, success, or compliance. However, you can use process information to assess your progress, provided you establish a standard or a criterion with which to compare that information.

A standard upon which to compare the process information can be established by using one or more of the following types of criteria:

- Performance criteria from a funder (e.g., CDC program announcement, foundation RFP);

- Criteria developed as part of the program planning and development process (e.g., SMART objectives, strategic plan);

- Criteria developed as part of the evaluation planning process (e.g., by an evaluator in consultation with program staff or a diverse group of stakeholders such as a subgroup of the tobacco control coalition).

Each of these approaches should be supported by scientific guidance of evidence-based programming such as *Best Practices for Comprehensive Tobacco Control Programs*,[1] *The Guide to Community Preventive Services*,[6] and *Communities of Excellence in Tobacco Control*.[7] In addition, such criteria should be reasonable within the local context.

To briefly illustrate how process indicators can be compared to hypothetical criteria, we present example inputs, activities, and outputs that were gathered through field interviews during full-day site visits with nine states, discussion groups with state tobacco control staff nationwide, and literature reviews. These are examples of the inputs, activities, and outputs identified as key elements of comprehensive tobacco use prevention and control programs.

The comparison of actual inputs, activities, and outputs (as measured through process evaluation) to established criteria can assist state and territorial tobacco control managers in:

- Identification of discrepancies between planned and actual implementation of the program or intervention;

- Identification of effective and ineffective implementation and management strategies; and,

- Improved understanding of whether and how program activities contribute to achieving desired short-term outcomes.

In **Exhibits 3-2, 3-3,** and **3-4,** we provide examples of how process information can inform decisions about programmatic issues such as these. It is very important to note that these are merely examples for you to consider in developing your own criteria and indicators, and they should not be considered as recommended by CDC for adoption.

Exhibit 3-2 lists example inputs, example criteria for measuring these against, and example indicators for measuring them.

Exhibit 3-2:   Inputs—Comparing Indicators to Criteria

Type of Input	Example Criteria	Example Input Indicators
Funding	CDC-recommended levels per *Best Practices* guidelines	Dollars allocated for each program component
Staffing	Required or recommended staffing as described in CDC funding opportunity announcement (FOA)	Actual staffing
Staff Skills	50% of staff will be trained in cultural competence and 85% will of those trained will assess the training as high quality	Percentage of staff trained in cultural competence, and percentage who assess training as high quality
Partnerships	75% of partners perceive the state as inclusive of their views in its planning and implementation	Survey/interview data on partners' perceptions of the degree to which the state is inclusive of their views in its planning and implementation

Specific community or statewide initiatives or programs will select activities that they feel best fit the population they want to address with the financial resources available, and with respect to political, social, and cultural considerations. Activities they might select appear in the first column of **Exhibit 3-3**. Please note that these activities may be carried out by NTCP grantees, partners collaborating with the grantees, or partners on their own.

For each activity implemented, outputs can also be measured. If output standards exist or are developed, you can compare actual outputs to expected outputs. Example activities with corresponding outputs, including example criteria and indicators for each, are listed in **Exhibit 3-3**. While **Exhibit 3-1** provides a description of some of these types of activities, the following criteria contain evaluative components. This ensures that the information gathered includes not only a description of the activity, but also an assessment of the quality of that activity. In the first example (i.e., counter-marketing), the output not only includes the percentage of the population reached, but also an assessment of the cultural appropriateness of the message.

In order to clarify how to understand and use **Exhibit 3-3**, the following example related to counter-marketing is provided.

> A state health department conducted an evaluation survey and found that compared to other groups, African-Americans were less likely to report having smoke-free home and automobile rules, and their children were more likely to be exposed to secondhand smoke. To address these disparities, the tobacco foundation in the state provided a grant to conduct a multi-channel counter-marketing campaign to influence knowledge, attitudes, and behaviors of African-Americans related to secondhand smoke exposure. Results of a process evaluation of the counter-marketing campaign showed that it was implemented in print and radio, and TV via public service announcements (PSAs) rather than paid spots. When planning the campaign, the state established the criteria that 75% of African-American adults will recall the campaign messages and perceive them to be appropriate for their community. In order to evaluate the effectiveness of the campaign, the state contracted with an evaluator to work with the local association of African-American churches to conduct an evaluation. Evaluation components included a brief written survey of a random sample and four discussion groups with church members. Results showed that 45% of those surveyed could recall the messages and that the messages were most frequently heard on the radio. Discussion group results with church members who had seen the campaign showed that 90% of them felt the messages were appropriate for their community. Consequently, the state determined that for the next counter-marketing campaign, they would not only implement the campaign using TV, radio and print, but that the emphasis would be on radio spots. Additionally, to evaluate outcomes, the state planned to include questions assessing exposure to the ads and changes in attitudes and behavior in a subsequent population-based evaluation survey.

In analogous fashion, you can compare information on program activities with criteria for understanding the capacity of interventions to identify and eliminate tobacco-related disparities. In **Exhibit 3-4,** we provide several examples of activity and output criteria and process indicators. Again, it is important to note that these are provided as illustrative examples only, and do not represent programmatic guidelines from CDC on inputs, activities, outputs, criteria, or indicators.

Introduction to Process Evaluation in Tobacco Use Prevention and Control

Exhibit 3-3: Activities and Outputs—Comparing Indicators to Criteria

Type of Activity	Activity		Output	
	Example Criteria	Example Indicators	Example Criteria	Example Indicators
Counter-marketing	Implementation of a culturally appropriate multi-channel media campaign (TV, radio, and print) encouraging African Americans to develop smoke-free home and automobile rules	Description of whether and how counter-advertising campaign is implemented	75% of African-American adults recall the campaign messages about secondhand smoke exposure in homes and automobiles and perceive them as appropriate for their community	Percentage of African-Americans that recall campaign messages and perceive them to be appropriate for their community
Policy and regulatory action	Collaboration with governmental agencies and partners to develop a comprehensive plan to carry out smoke-free law implementation (e.g., signage, educating businesses)	Description of process used to develop plan (e.g., identification of stakeholders, steps taken to develop plan)	Quality written comprehensive implementation plan completed in collaboration with appropriate government agencies and partners	Appropriate external secondhand smoke policy experts assess implementation plan as high quality
	Minimum of 6 earned media spots, quarterly press conferences, and press releases on current policy and regulatory issues (e.g., taxation, secondhand smoke policy)	Number of media spots, press conferences/press releases, and topics addressed	Quarterly newspaper articles and editorials as a result of press conferences and press releases	Frequency of articles and editorials that reference materials or information provided in the press release and/or press conference
Community mobilization	Provision of appropriate, timely and useful technical assistance to all local partners	Description of whether and how technical assistance is provided to local partners	85% of local partners assess technical assistance as appropriate, timely, and useful	Percentage of local partners that assess technical assistance as appropriate, timely and useful
School-based prevention	Complete an assessment of the existence of and perceived compliance with tobacco-free school policies	Description of whether tobacco-free school policies are in place and perceptions of compliance	75% of school districts respond to the survey of tobacco-free school policies and data are used to develop an action plan to increase school district coverage	Response rate to assessment and action plan to increase school coverage

24

Section 3—Information Elements Central to Process Evaluation

Type of Activity	Activity		Output	
	Example Criteria	Example Indicators	Example Criteria	Example Indicators
Partnership development	Collaborative relationships will be established with each CDC funded National Network to reduce tobacco related disparities with their respective priority population groups	Number of agreements to work with the National Networks	As a result of each collaboration, one strategy and two opportunities to reach and impact each priority population will be identified and assessed as culturally competent by priority population representatives	Identified strategies and opportunities assessed by priority population representatives as culturally competent
Strategic plan to address disparities	A group composed of appropriate and diverse stakeholders will work to develop a disparities strategic plan	Evidence of involvement of stakeholders from priority populations in development of plan	A disparities strategic plan will be developed and incorporated into the overall strategic plan, along with implementation strategies	Overall strategic plan, including disparities plan and implementation strategies
Knowledge integration	Using knowledge about tobacco-related disparities, two culturally competent interventions will be implemented with priority populations	Priority populations and interventions identified	Two tailored population-based interventions implemented as designed reaching 40% of the identified priority populations	Evaluation will show implementation of the interventions as designed (i.e., fidelity) and percentage of priority population reached
Surveillance	Develop and implement surveillance systems that are able to identify tobacco-related disparities	Description of whether and how knowledge, attitudes, and behavior of specific populations can be sampled and estimated	Data on two specific populations are collected and analyzed	Evidence that data systems describing tobacco-related knowledge, attitudes, and behavior meet professional standards
Evaluation	Conduct evaluation of quitline promotional campaign to reach rural populations	Evaluation of promotional campaign conducted	Evaluation completed and used to inform decisions about how to increase rural populations' utilization of the quitline	Assessment of whether and how evaluation results were used by decision makers to inform decisions about the quitline

25

Introduction to Process Evaluation in Tobacco Use Prevention and Control

---

CASE EXAMPLE: *PROGRAM STRUCTURE AND COMPONENTS*

Implementation of the Henry J. Kaiser Family Foundation's Community Health Promotion Grant Program

In 1986, the Kaiser Family Foundation initiated the Community Health Promotion Grant Program to help communities develop health interventions in one or more targeted health areas. Funded sites in 11 communities in the western United States received grants of up to $450,000 and were given great flexibility in developing and implementing intervention activities that were appropriate for their communities. Grantees were asked to: (1) establish a coalition with a broad range of community agencies and organizations, (2) conduct a formal needs assessment, and (3) address one or more of the five targeted health issues.

How process evaluation was helpful:

Because grantees were given latitude in developing coalitions and implementing interventions, it was critical that the research team could gather information to describe the program in each community. The type of information collected on the program and target area included type of location (urban/suburban/rural), target area population, community population demographics, sponsoring agency, health target areas, primary intervention audience, impetus for the program, and a description of the primary interventions.

Advantages for you:

Findings from this component of the process evaluation revealed considerable variation across sites, in terms of both the interventions used and the target populations. Information on program structure and components in the various sites was critical to interpreting other findings from the process and outcome evaluations.

SOURCE: Wickizer TM, Wagner E, Cheadle A, Pearson D, Beery W, Maeser J, et al. Implementation of the Henry J. Kaiser Family Foundation's Community Health Promotion Grant Program: A process evaluation. *Milbank Quarterly* 1998;76(1):121–47.

CASE EXAMPLE: *THEORY AND FIDELITY*

New York Statewide School Tobacco Policy Review

Enactment of the federal Pro-Children's Act of 1994 and other public health laws has prompted schools to create policies that address the tobacco issue. However, little was known about the quality of these resulting school policies. To assess the quality of all New York schools' tobacco policies, the New York State Education Department (NYSED) commissioned a systematic review. NYSED designated the Statewide Center for Healthy Schools to lead the review of tobacco policies submitted by all New York school districts between April and August 2001.

How process evaluation was helpful:

The Center developed a policy rubric using two guides: *Fit, Healthy, and Ready to Learn* and the *School Health Index*. The rubric assessed five policy components including (1) Developing, Overseeing, and Communicating the Policy (2) Purpose and Goals, (3) Tobacco-Free Environments, (4) Tobacco Use Prevention Education, and (5) Assistance to Overcome Tobacco Addictions. In total, 471 tobacco policies were reviewed using this rubric. Results demonstrated that overall, policy scores were low.

Advantages for you:

The assessment demonstrated that many school districts had policies that did not provide tobacco-free environments for students and that additional technical assistance should be provided to assist schools in developing and enforcing effective policies consistent with CDC guidelines. In many cases it appeared that tobacco policies were developed by outside counsel with little consideration given to developing practical tobacco policies using input from key stakeholders and/or the larger community. These results prompted increased efforts to provide information, training, and technical assistance to the school districts to help improve their tobacco policies.

SOURCE: Stephens YD, English G. A statewide school tobacco policy review: Process, results, and implications. *Journal of School Health* 2002;72(8):334–338.

CASE EXAMPLE: *COLLABORATIONS AND PARTNERSHIPS*

Elimination of Secondhand Smoke through the Seattle and King County Smoke-Free Housing Initiative

There is no safe level of exposure to secondhand smoke. Washington State law protects King County from exposure in public places and the workplace; the greatest exposure thus occurs in the home. Striving for a complete smoke-free policy means that smoking is prohibited in all private units of multi-unit housing, all indoor common areas, and in outdoor areas, including all patios, porches, and decks and anywhere from which smoke can drift to the inside.

How process evaluation was helpful:

The King County Tobacco Prevention Program has identified two strategies to promote smoke-free policies in housing: regulatory and voluntary.

The regulatory strategy includes changing zoning codes to prohibit smoking in multifamily residential units in King County and for Public Health to name secondhand smoke as a nuisance under Washington's nuisance law. Through an action of the Board of Health, smoke-free multi-unit housing could become a regulation. Partnering with development and management companies to demonstrate the value and viability of smoke-free housing is one tactic to influence regulation, as well as working through the policy-development channels within the County's health department.

The voluntary strategy is to assist property managers, landlords, and condominium boards to introduce smoke-free policies with education and technical assistance and to empower tenants to work with the property decision-makers. Tactics include increasing tenant awareness, using targeted and broad-scale media, conducting outreach with the largest owners of multi-unit housing, and partnering with rental associations to provide education and tools.

Each tactic contains specific measurables (e.g., number of partnerships, training attendees, quantity and quality of media). Collecting this process evaluation information by monitoring progress made will help determine which activities are fruitful and worth more investment, and which goals may need a different approach.

Advantages for you:

Careful monitoring of each of a program's intermediate objectives, with corresponding recording of achievements -- such as zoning code changes, number of units smoke-free -- enables you to know which tactics better lead to accomplishment of desired outcomes.

SOURCE: Public Health, Seattle and King County Smoke Free Housing Initiative, Tobacco Prevention Program (Brochure, 2006).

4. MANAGING PROCESS EVALUATION

As noted in the Introduction, there is no single right way to design and conduct process evaluations. The following chapter provides an overview of critical evaluation standards, and practical procedures for managing evaluation.[11] These fundamental components are intended to provide a foundation for effective utilization-focused, participatory evaluation design and implementation. Information on managing evaluation has been included to provide practical guidance on clarifying roles and responsibilities as you work with consultants and stakeholders throughout the evaluation process.

Although the following 10-step process identifies general stages of the evaluation process, clarifies roles, and suggests realistic time horizons for completing each stage of an evaluation, the process is not prescriptive regarding the methods and content of the evaluation. The model is flexible: it can be adapted to the local context, and used for both process and outcome evaluations. While it may not be necessary for every evaluation study, a primary benefit of the process is that it ensures that program staff and evaluators work together with stakeholders.

4.1 Managing Process Evaluation: A 10-Step Process

Although the conceptual information provided in the previous sections is useful in framing and directing an approach to evaluation, it does not provide practical guidance on how to apply these concepts in the day-to-day management of evaluation. Program managers often ask questions such as these:

- How do you manage an evaluation of a large state government program?
- Why have an evaluation advisory group? Who should be on it?
- How do you coordinate an evaluation of programs at the community level?
- What are the defined roles of evaluation staff and stakeholders?
- How can the program manager work effectively with the evaluation staff and stakeholders?
- How do you identify which staff should be involved?
- How do you work effectively with external evaluation consultants?

4.1.1 Purpose: Why Use the 10-Step Process for Managing Evaluation?

One issue faced by tobacco control managers in conducting evaluation is identifying an appropriate evaluator. It can be challenging to identify an evaluator who is comfortable with a participatory model for conducting evaluation and accepts the Joint Committee Evaluation Standards (See Section 4.2). This process has been designed as a way of operationalizing the utilization-focused approach to evaluation, which posits that the primary criterion for judging an evaluation should be its use.[8] As noted in the Introduction of this manual, process evaluations can be used for program improvement, monitoring, and accountability. However, to ensure that information collected, analyzed, and reported meets the needs of all stakeholders, you should work with the people who will be using this information from the beginning of the evaluation process, and focus on how they will use it.

The 10-step process for managing evaluation helps program managers and evaluators address questions like those posed above. It is a practical and usable approach that clearly defines the roles and responsibilities of the program manager (or designee) and the evaluator as they work closely with an advisory group of primary intended users and stakeholders.[12] This process was field tested for five years and provides a practical approach to process evaluation.[12]

The process involves an evaluation advisory group, an evaluation facilitator (typically the program manager or designee), and the evaluator (internal staff or an external consultant). The 10-step process builds evaluation capacity in program staff by creating a common understanding of evaluation and a systematic process for designing and implementing it.

It also enhances the evaluator's ability to engage stakeholders and collaboratively plan and implement a utilization-focused evaluation.[10] The process increases the likelihood of the evaluator producing a useful report by working with the evaluation advisory group to conceptualize the study, develop the evaluation questions, and assist in the interpretation of the data.

4.1.2 Roles of the Advisory Group, Evaluation Facilitator, and Evaluator

An overview of the roles of the evaluation advisory group, the evaluation facilitator, and the evaluator in the 10-Step process is presented below. Appendix C provides additional details on the evaluation advisory group, including the benefits of establishing one, selection of group members, and further details on the responsibilities of the advisory group.

Role of the evaluation advisory group: The advisory group's function is to provide input throughout the evaluation, to help the evaluator think through various program issues, to review drafts of the evaluation plan and data collection instruments, to provide insights into the collected data, and to make recommendations based on the evaluation's findings. The group's role is a reflective one, not one of making final decisions about the evaluation's design, implementation, or final report. In addition, the advisory group provides insights into the social and/or political context of the program being evaluated, which often accounts for the variation in how programs are implemented.

Role of the evaluation facilitator: The evaluation facilitator plays a central role throughout the 10-step process. In general, facilitators manage the relationship between the evaluation advisory group and the evaluator, help to select an appropriate evaluation design, garner organizational and political support to implement the evaluation, provide technical and logistical assistance, and facilitate the use of the evaluation results among primary intended users and program stakeholders. Managing these relationships is crucial to ensure that the input and feedback provided by the advisory group is reflected in the evaluation design and implementation.

The evaluation facilitator also plays a critical role in building organizational capacity to conduct evaluation by identifying and selecting an appropriate evaluator, as well as working with the evaluator to provide a comprehensive introduction to key evaluation concepts, as needed, to the advisory group.

Either the program manager or a designee who is integrally involved in the programmatic aspects of the intervention and/or program should serve as the evaluation facilitator. The evaluator should not serve as both evaluation facilitator and evaluator because it will likely diminish the benefits of the 10-step process and will increase the risk that the evaluation is designed without meaningful programmatic insight, which could ultimately reduce capacity for evaluation and negatively impact use of evaluation results.

Role of the evaluator: The evaluator is responsible for making final decisions on the evaluation's design, data collection instruments, data collection methods and procedures, data analysis, and writing of the final report. While there may be issues that the evaluator needs to negotiate with the advisory group, the evaluator is ultimately responsible for carrying out the evaluation in an effective, ethical, and professional manner.

4.1.3 Stages and Steps of the 10-Step Process

The 10-step evaluation process provides a protocol for participants to follow that outlines each step in four stages: groundwork, formalization, implementation, and utilization. An overview of the four stages of the 10-step process and the suggested timeline for a 12-month evaluation are presented in **Exhibit 4-1**. The timeline can be adjusted to the local context as needed. For example, when evaluating a two-year project, the implementation phase could take longer than is presented in **Exhibit 4-1**.

Exhibit 4-1: Overview of the 10-Step Process for Managing Evaluation

Stage	Steps
I. Groundwork In this stage, the evaluation plan is drafted, with attention to how the evaluation process and findings will be used in decisions about policy and programmatic modification or termination. The study's purpose, questions, and methods is determined during this stage.	1–3 (Approximately 11 weeks)
II. Formalization In this stage, the formal agreements, supporting infrastructure, and details of implementation are negotiated and agreed on. This stage includes development of the proposal and data collection instruments and compliance with IRB policies (and OMB for federal institutions), if applicable.	4–5 (Approximately 11 weeks)
III. Implementation In this stage, the program evaluation is conducted and data collection and preliminary analyses are completed. Special attention is given to early findings and possible recommendations. Then, a draft report is prepared and there is further formalization of the study's findings and potential resulting recommendations. The draft report is reviewed by the evaluation advisory group, and the report is finalized with their input.	6–8 (Approximately 23 weeks)
IV. Utilization In this stage, the findings are translated into decisions for action.	9–10 (Approximately 7 weeks)

Detailed information on all ten steps of the process, as well as the responsibilities and activities of the evaluation facilitator and the evaluator for each step, are presented in **Exhibit 4-2**. The responsibilities and activities of the evaluation advisory group at various steps throughout the process are also specified.

Exhibit 4-2: Steps and Staff Responsibilities in the 10-Step Process

STAGE I. GROUNDWORK		
	Role of Evaluation Facilitator	**Role of Evaluator**
STEP 1:	Identify evaluation project and evaluator	
a.	Meets with key program staff to identify priority evaluation topic	
b.	Identifies external consultant or in-house evaluator	
STEP 2:	Conference call or meeting with key staff and evaluator	
a.	Schedules conference call or meeting with key staff and evaluator to discuss basic information needed to plan the evaluation (e.g., purpose; logic model; identification of intended users, uses, and stakeholders)	Participates in conference call or meeting
STEP 3:	Collaboration with advisory group to plan the evaluation	
a.	Identifies evaluation advisory group	Assists with identification of a diverse advisory group
b.	Schedules meeting or call with the advisory group and the evaluator (minimum of 2 hours) to get input on: • purpose/uses of the evaluation • users of the evaluation • evaluation questions • methodologies • political considerations	Participates in meeting
STAGE II. FORMALIZATION		
STEP 4:	Proposal and data collection instruments are drafted, distributed, and reviewed	
a.		Drafts proposal and data collection instruments (e.g., written surveys, telephone surveys, personal/group interviews)
b.	Reviews draft proposal and data collection instruments with program manager and recommends changes if necessary; approves proposal, instruments, and plan for participant protection	
c.	Once approved by program manager, distributes plans to evaluation advisory group for 2-week review	
d.	Collects feedback on proposal and data collection instruments from evaluation advisory group and forwards to evaluator	

(Continued)

Exhibit 4-2:   Steps and Staff Responsibilities in the 10-Step Process (continued)

STAGE II. FORMALIZATION (continued)		
	Role of Evaluation Facilitator	**Role of Evaluator**
STEP 5:	Proposal and data collection instruments revised, finalized, and submitted for IRB approval; contract signed if using external evaluator	
a.	Approves final proposal and data collection instruments with program manager	Finalizes proposal and data collection instrument/works to comply with IRB process
b.	Ensures appropriate staff sign proposal, which is attached to contract if using an external evaluator	Signs proposal
STAGE III. IMPLEMENTATION		
STEP 6:	Data collection, entry, and analysis	
a.		Collects, enters, and analyzes data; prepares preliminary findings; sends findings to evaluation facilitator
b.	Reviews preliminary findings/shares with program manager	
STEP 7:	Preliminary findings are shared with evaluation advisory group	
a.	Distributes findings to evaluation advisory group	
b.	Schedules call or meeting with evaluation advisory group to discuss findings and identify format for reporting findings	Participates in evaluation advisory group meeting
STEP 8:	Draft report prepared, distributed, reviewed, and finalized	
a.		Prepares draft report
b.	Reviews report and shares with program manager	
c.	Once approved by program manager, distributes to advisory group for 2-week review	
d.	Collects feedback from advisory group and forwards to evaluator	
e.		Finalizes report
STAGE IV. UTILIZATION		
STEP 9:	Meeting to wrap up evaluation study and discuss utilization of findings and dissemination of report(s)	
a.	Schedules meeting with evaluator to review the evaluation process and discuss how the evaluation can be used, and if appropriate, the development of the next evaluation	Participates in meeting
b.	Disseminates report to intended users/stakeholders and others	

(Continued)

Exhibit 4-2: **Steps and Staff Responsibilities in the 10-Step Process (continued)**

STAGE IV. UTILIZATION (continued)		
	Role of Evaluation Facilitator	**Role of Evaluator**
STEP 10:	Development of action plan for use of the evaluation	
a.	Develops action plan with program manager for implementation and monitoring	Participates as appropriate
b.	Continues evaluation process; targets area for evaluation from first year or identifies new priority topic for evaluation	

4.1.4 Further Guidance on Implementing the 10-Step Process

Considerations for Stage I: Stage I activities focus on engaging the evaluation advisory group and developing a feasible evaluation plan. However, the very first step is to identify exactly what program or intervention will be evaluated. Tobacco control programs are complex, multi-component systems that include community coalitions, policy directives, mass media campaigns, and telephone quitlines, among other activities. The following criteria will help you identify projects or program activities that will increase your ability to complete a useful evaluation:

- The selected program/intervention should be significant and of importance to tobacco use prevention and control. It should be of sufficient importance that the process evaluation and report will be seriously reviewed in policy and program decisions.

- It should provide practical questions to address.

- Staff should be motivated to do process evaluation on the topic.

- The process evaluation must provide data that address the questions being asked by the program staff/stakeholders.

- There must be agreement that the program can be evaluated within the agreed upon cost and time frame.

- The process evaluation should be sensitive to the interests of a wide range of tobacco use prevention and control stakeholders.

- When possible, data should be collected that will allow decisions to be made on different levels (e.g., program decisions, management decisions).

- The data produced must be useful for decision making.

If needed, evaluation advisory group members should be provided with a brief introduction to the fundamentals of evaluation prior to the initial advisory group meeting. Two potential resources include *Introduction to Program Evaluation in Comprehensive Tobacco Control Programs*[2] and *Utilization-Focused Evaluation*.[8] Orienting advisory group members in this way will foster their participation in the process and enhance the capacity for evaluation. It will also prepare advisory group members to assist with identifying primary evaluation uses, prioritizing key evaluation questions, and assessing appropriate data collection methods. Ideally, the evaluation facilitator and the evaluator will participate in this introduction as a way to build rapport with advisory group members.

The initial advisory group meeting (Step 3b) is a critical milestone in the evaluation. Effectively engaging the advisory group in the evaluation planning will set the stage for continued success throughout the evaluation process. Careful preparation should be made to ensure the active participation of all advisory group members in critically assessing the core components of the evaluation plan.

One challenge that often arises during the first evaluation advisory group meeting is that more evaluation questions are identified than can be answered within the timeframe and resources available to conduct the study. When this occurs, advisory group members must prioritize the identified evaluation questions. Failure to do so can result in an inability to adequately answer the most useful evaluation questions within resource limitations.

Considerations for Stage II: Stage II activities include formalizing the process evaluation plan. Ideally, the final plan will be included as part of the statement of work in the formal contract if an outside evaluator is used. However, you may find it necessary to finalize the evaluator contract prior to beginning any work on the evaluation. If so, it is best to be as explicit as possible in the request for proposals and the statement of work with the evaluator regarding the use of a participatory process to be used when developing and completing the evaluation. Explicitly telling the evaluator that it is required to effectively engage primary evaluation users throughout the evaluation project will help avoid frustration. Too often, contractors work independently of the program staff and primary intended evaluation users, and may fail to meet the program evaluation standards (See Section 4.2.1); and this often results in a final report with little to no information useful for program improvement, monitoring, or accountability purposes.

Considerations for Stage III: Stage III, evaluation implementation, takes the longest amount of time to complete. Implementation involves data collection and analyses, as well as meetings with the evaluation advisory group to help interpret the findings. This latter component is critical because the advisory group will have valuable insight into programmatic issues that drive the results.

The evaluation advisory group will also play a critical role in determining the best format for reporting results that will be used in program decision making. Historically, evaluations culminate in a lengthy final report that uses standard scientific research principles to report methodology, findings, and conclusions. Unfortunately, this formal report often becomes a barrier to practical use of the evaluation information. You should work with the evaluation advisory group to identify the most effective ways to report evaluation information and the optimal timeline for release of this information to overcome this barrier, recognizing that multiple reports may be needed for different audiences. The format and timeline for reporting process evaluation information should be driven by the primary purpose and planned uses of the evaluation. For example, process information collected to improve the program must be available quickly to maximize its use in making midcourse changes and improvements. Clarifying the form and structure for communicating evaluation information will be an iterative process based on the changing needs of the primary evaluation users. Because advisory group members represent the primary users of the evaluation information, the advisory group is the best source of guidance on form and function of the summaries within the given context of the program. Following are some alternative formats for reporting evaluation results:[13]

Section 4—Managing Process Evaluation

- Short communication (memo, fax, e-mail)
- Personal discussions with stakeholders
- Interim/progress reports
- Executive summaries
- Chart essays
- Verbal presentations
- Newsletters, bulletins, and brochures
- Videotape presentations
- Poster presentations
- Public meetings
- News media communication

Considerations for Stage IV: Stage IV includes utilization of evaluation information and dissemination of evaluation findings to primary stakeholders. During this stage, evaluation findings and recommendations are translated into implementation decisions.[12] Note that creation of the dissemination plan is a distinct process from development of an evaluation plan.

Tailoring the 10-step process: The process was designed to be completed in approximately 12 months. However, the process is adaptable to local context and to studies of different lengths. For example, a study can be implemented for 6, 12, or 18 months using the same framework by adjusting the time frames for each stage.

This process can also be used with an expert panel that is convened to identify the evidence base for the program, and to provide guidance to the development of a logic model. The inclusion of select expert panel members on the advisory committee can contribute a valuable perspective to practical concerns such as evaluation questions, methods, and use.

4.2   The Program Evaluation Standards and Protecting Participants in Evaluation Research

4.2.1 The Program Evaluation Standards

The Program Evaluation Standards of the Joint Committee on Standards for Evaluation[14] outline a set of utility, feasibility, propriety, and accuracy standards that will help you to develop and implement an ethical, useful process evaluation that makes the best use of limited resources. (See Appendix B for more information.) As you identify evaluators to assist with the design and completion of your process evaluation, you should make sure that they are familiar with and hold themselves accountable to these professional standards. Additionally, when the 10-Step Process for Managing Evaluation is used, the evaluation facilitator, evaluator, and evaluation advisory group should be familiar with the standards and agree that the evaluation will conform to them.

The standards are designed to ensure that the evaluation follows four overarching principles:

1. *Utility*: The evaluation will serve the information needs of intended users.

2. *Feasibility*: The evaluation will be realistic, prudent, diplomatic, and frugal.

3. *Accuracy*: The evaluation will reveal and convey technically adequate information about the features that determine worth or merit of the program being evaluated.

4. *Propriety*: The evaluation will be conducted legally, ethically, and with due regard for the welfare of those involved in the evaluation, as well as those affected by its results.

4.2.2 Protecting Participants in Evaluation Research

Investigators conducting research studies that require contact with human subjects (e.g., surveys, focus group discussions) typically must receive Institutional Review Board (IRB) approval. However, a program evaluation intended to gather information solely for improving that program (as opposed to producing generalizable knowledge) is not necessarily considered research. Non-research studies do not necessarily need IRB review. Whether IRB review will be required depends on the local context. Program managers should check with their institution's IRB before starting evaluation studies to determine whether IRB approval will be required. IRB reviews take time, so this determination should be made as early as possible.

IRBs review study protocols to ensure that they comply with standards for protection of human subjects.[2] When IRB approval is required by an institution, the requirement also pertains to the institution's contractors on the study. If an institution lacks an IRB, it is possible to request review by an IRB at another institution. IRBs that are registered as agreeing to follow federal policy on human research subject protection are listed at http://ohrp.cit.nih.gov/search/asearch.asp#23ASUR.

Federal government institutions are also subject to requirements of the Paperwork Reduction Act. This Act prohibits federal entities from engaging in systematic data collection from more than nine individuals or institutions without approval from the U.S. Office of Management and Budget (OMB). This requirement applies regardless of whether the information is being collected for evaluation or research purposes.

---

[2] For more information, see http://www.hhs.gov/ohrp/policy/index.html.

4.3 Choosing a Process Evaluation Design (Methodology)

The evaluator works with the advisory group to select the best data collection method for the given purpose of the process evaluation. Evaluation data can be quantitative (i.e., quantifiable, numerically expressed information), qualitative (i.e., information in a narrative format), or a combination of both. Quantitative methods generally use standardized instruments to collect data, which are transferred into numerical values and analyzed using statistical methods. Collection and analysis of quantitative data is often perceived to be more objective. However, quantitative data often lack the richness of information provided by qualitative methods.

Qualitative methods are appropriate for the collection of detailed descriptions of processes and for program accountability, monitoring, and improvement. Specifically, process data can provide detailed information on how a program operates, whether it is operating as expected, and what program elements are more (or less) successful. Formative evaluations focusing on program improvement often use process data.[15] Qualitative methods typically provide stronger evaluation tools (1) when there is uncertainty as to why a program component or intervention is or is not working or (2) when the evaluator is searching for unidentified variables. Open-ended qualitative data, unrestricted by predetermined categories, are often used in process evaluations because these data can provide detailed answers to complex issues not yet understood by the evaluator or program manager. This type of data collection method "emphasizes understanding, rather than precise measurement, of events"; it is a dynamic process where evidence can be gathered using multiple perspectives.[16] The data collection is geared toward understanding processes affecting program staff and participants.

Regardless of the data collection method used, the evaluator needs to take the following six issues into account when identifying which measurement tools to use:[9]

1. Type of data collection required.

2. Frequency of data collection.

3. Persons responsible for data collection.

4. Reliability (degree to which an instrument provides a consistent rating) and validity (degree to which an instrument measures what it is supposed to) of the data collection measures.

5. Cost.

6. Potential burden to participants and staff members.

The evaluator should discuss these issues with the program manager to identify the most appropriate data collection tool(s).[3] Some common qualitative research methods used in process evaluation are:[17]

- Case studies;

- Structured or semi-structured interviews with or self-administered surveys of program stakeholders to gather information on program activity facilitators and barriers;

---

[3]For additional ideas regarding evaluation methodology for tobacco programs, and for links to websites with practical evaluation tools, consult the Tobacco Technical Assistance Consortium – www.ttac.org.

- Focus groups with participants, staff, or informants to generate information on the program's design or suggestions for program improvement;

- Direct observation to record participant and project staff behavior during an intervention; and

- Recorded reviews of minutes from program meetings, progress reports from subcontractors, self-report inventories, diaries, or project archives.

A variety of tools can be used to analyze and interpret qualitative data. Two commonly used software programs[4] are NVivo7[18] and ATLAS.ti.[19] For example, ATLAS.ti allows the analysis of electronic text, images (e.g., scans of handwritten notes), video (e.g., television counter-marketing advertisements), and audio (e.g., radio counter-marketing, digitized interviews).

Two quantitative research methods are:

- Conducting surveys to measure participants' understanding of the program or identify the source of a program's problem; and

- Tracking data in the form of record reviews to count the number of items distributed or collected, such as program logs measuring the number of brochures distributed, smoke-free home pledges distributed/received, number of people contacted or reached by the project, and number of training sessions held.

As you consider data collection method(s), it is critical to involve the evaluation advisory group to determine which methods are feasible. The evaluator should act as a consultant to ensure that the evaluation methodology is as strong as possible; successful programs cannot be proven effective without a defensible evaluation.

Note that much process evaluation information comes from the documents and records that programs typically create as a part of normal operations. It is rarely necessary to construct completely new data collection procedures in order to do process evaluation, even though it may be necessary to take steps to ensure that existing data collection procedures are formalized for accuracy and completeness.

So, for example, information on inputs may appear in descriptive materials, approved budgets, board minutes, inter-agency agreements (which specify partners and roles), and other documents. Information on the types of activities for programs will often appear in strategic plans, work plans, staff logs, and inter-agency agreements. Outputs are typically documented through work logs, participation records, and sometimes expenditure records and accounting reports.

---

[4]Use of trade names is for identification only and does not imply endorsement by the Centers for Disease Control and Prevention or the U.S. Department of Health and Human Services.

4.4 Process Evaluation—Beyond a Single Study

You may use the steps and techniques described in this section for a single evaluation. However, you will most likely conduct multiple process evaluations, either simultaneously or sequentially. This will require ongoing commitment to evaluation (process and outcome) and ongoing allocation of resources. Optimally, it will also include ongoing use of evaluation information for the purposes of program monitoring, program improvement, development of effective program models, and accountability (as described in Section 2).

Participatory models of evaluation that engage stakeholders to serve in advisory roles (like the 10-step process described in Section 4.1) enhance the use and applicability of evaluation information.[20] The participatory approach builds an appreciation, knowledge, and acceptance of evaluation among those people and organizations that participate in the evaluation process. This, in turn, encourages the use of evaluation information in everyday program decision making. As you do more and more participatory evaluations, using the process just described, you will increase the capacity of your organization both to carry out effective program evaluation and to use evaluation findings routinely.[21]

You may find it useful to have someone in your organization focus beyond the process, completion, and timely use of any single evaluation study. This person or group could review what each discrete study has accomplished, build on the learning acquired from each study, and work to create and sustain organizational structures and processes to implement and use evaluation. Evaluation capacity building is a worthwhile process to increase the likelihood of quality evaluation becoming a regular and routine part of your organization's work.[21]

5. CONCLUSION

Process evaluation is an important part of identifying ways to improve your program, monitor program implementation, build effective program models, and demonstrate accountability. Used in coordination with outcome evaluation, process evaluation enables you to better focus your time and resources where they will have the greatest benefit. In the ever-changing landscape of tobacco use prevention and control, systematic collection of process information over time will help you efficiently modify program components and activities as needed. This ability to effectively compensate for changing external environments and priorities will increase your capacity to address the health consequences of tobacco use and to justify program funding.

The remainder of this document contains references, a glossary of terms, and five appendices covering CDC's framework for program evaluation (Appendix A); the program evaluation standards of the Joint Committee on Standards for Evaluation (Appendix B); detailed information on purpose, selection, and role of the evaluation advisory group (Appendix C); and examples of evaluation questions related to the Center for Tobacco Policy Research's logic model (Appendix D).

GLOSSARY OF TERMS

Activities: The actual events or actions that take place as a part of a program.

Evaluation plan: A written document describing the overall evaluation approach or design. The plan describes what will be done, how it will be done, who will do it, when it will be done, why the evaluation is being conducted, and how the findings will likely be used.

Indicator: A specific, observable measure of an input, activity, output, or outcome of a program.

Infrastructure: All the components necessary to conduct an evaluation (e.g., experienced staff, adequate funding).

Inputs: Resources used to plan and set up a program.

Logic model: A systematic and visual way to present the perceived relationships among the resources you have to operate the program, the activities you plan to do, and the results you hope to achieve.

Objectives: Quantifiable statements describing the results to be achieved and the manner in which these results will be achieved. Objectives should be specific, measurable, achievable, relevant, and time-bound.

Outputs: The direct products of program activities; immediate measures of what the program did.

Outcomes: The results of program operations or activities; the effects triggered by the program, for example, policy or environmental changes at the state, community, or organizational level. At the individual level, outcomes might include changes in knowledge, skills, and attitudes or changes in behaviors such as tobacco use.

Outcome evaluation: The systematic collection of information to assess the impact of a program, present conclusions about the program's merit or worth, and make recommendations about future program direction or improvement.

Priority population: A specific population experiencing tobacco-related disparities that your program has identified for focused programmatic efforts.

Process evaluation: The systematic collection of information to document and assess how a program is implemented and operates. This information can help determine whether the program is being implemented as designed and can be used to improve the delivery and efficiency of the program.

Program evaluation: The systematic collection of information on a program's inputs, activities, and outputs, as well as the program's context and other key characteristics.

Reach: The absolute number, proportion, and representativeness of persons who are exposed to or participate in a given program or intervention. Representativeness refers to whether participants have characteristics that reflect the target population.

Social Ecological Model: A framework for understanding health behavior change. There are five levels at which change can occur: individual, interpersonal, organizational, community, and society.

Stakeholder: The persons or organizations that have a vested interest in what will be learned from an evaluation and what will be done with the information.[2]

Surveillance: The monitoring of tobacco-related behaviors, attitudes, and health outcomes at regular intervals of time.

Utility: The extent to which an evaluation produces reports that are disseminated to relevant audiences, inform program decisions, and have a beneficial effect.

Utilization-focused evaluation: A process for making decisions about critical evaluation issues, including purpose, design, and type of data to collect. The process involves collaboration with an identified group of primary users to determine their intended uses of evaluation findings.[8]

APPENDIX A:
CDC'S FRAMEWORK FOR PROGRAM EVALUATION[4]

Step 1: Engage stakeholders. The first step of the Framework involves identifying and engaging stakeholders to ensure that the perspectives and needs of the primary users of evaluation information are taken into account. Stakeholders are those people who have a vested interest in what will be learned from the evaluation and how the evaluation findings will be used. Stakeholders may include those involved in program operations, those participating in or affected by the program, and other primary users of the evaluation. The level of stakeholder involvement will vary from program to program; for example, stakeholders may provide input to the evaluator, they may help design the evaluation, and/or they may help collect the evaluation data.

Step 2: Describe the program. Describing the program helps to ensure that all parties agree on the definition and purpose of the program before undertaking an evaluation. A clear program description helps articulate program goals and objectives and facilitates comparisons with similar programs. A complete program description should include need, expected effects, activities, resources, stage of development, context, and logic model.

Step 3: Focus the evaluation. Focusing the evaluation involves working with stakeholders to prioritize evaluation questions and ensure that the evaluation design adheres to the standards for evaluation while making the most efficient use of time and resources. The key areas to consider when focusing the evaluation include purpose, users, uses, questions, methods, and agreements.

Step 4: Gather credible evidence. All information collected to conduct the evaluation must be useful, credible, and relevant to the key stakeholders and should provide a well-rounded assessment of the program to ensure that the evaluation addresses the program's key purposes. Credible evaluation evidence helps ensure the utility of the findings and the applicability for stakeholders and others interested in learning from the evaluation. To enhance credibility, carefully consider the indicators, data sources, quality, quantity, and logistics of gathering evidence. Balancing the accuracy and feasibility of evaluation data often becomes a challenge that should be addressed in collaboration with key stakeholders.

Step 5: Justify conclusions. The evaluation conclusions should be clearly linked to the evidence gathered during the program evaluation. Given their critical understanding of the context of the program, key stakeholders should play a primary role in interpreting evaluation evidence that will justify the evaluation conclusions. Justification of conclusions requires close adherence to standards. This step also includes analysis and synthesis of evaluation evidence, informed interpretation and judgment by key stakeholders, and development of recommendations to inform program decision makers.

Step 6: Ensure use and lessons learned. Effective evaluation requires time, effort, and resources. Given these investments, it is critical that the evaluation findings be disseminated appropriately and used to inform decision making and action. Once again, key stakeholders can provide critical information about the form, function, and distribution of evaluation findings to maximize their use.

APPENDIX B:
DETAILED LIST OF THE JOINT COMMITTEE ON STANDARDS FOR EVALUATION: THE PROGRAM EVALUATION STANDARDS[14]

Propriety Standards

The propriety standards are intended to ensure that an evaluation will be conducted legally, ethically, and with due regard for the welfare of those involved in the evaluation, as well as those affected by its results.

P1 Service orientation: Evaluations should be designed to assist organizations to address and effectively serve the needs of the full range of targeted participants.

P2 Formal agreements: Obligations of the formal parties to an evaluation (i.e., what is to be done, how, by whom, when) should be agreed to in writing, so that these parties are obligated to adhere to all conditions of the agreement or formally renegotiate commitments.

P3 Rights of human subjects: Evaluations should be designed and conducted to respect and protect the rights and welfare of human subjects.

P4 Human interactions: Evaluators should respect human dignity and worth in their interactions with other persons associated with an evaluation, so that participants are not threatened or harmed.

P5 Complete and fair assessment: The evaluation should be complete and fair in its examination and recording of strengths and weaknesses of the program being evaluated so that strengths can be built on and problem areas addressed.

P6 Disclosure of findings: The formal parties to an evaluation should ensure that the full set of evaluation findings, along with pertinent limitations, are made accessible to the persons affected by the evaluation and any others with expressed legal rights to receive the results.

P7 Conflict of interest: Conflict of interest should be dealt with openly and honestly so that it does not compromise the evaluation processes and results.

P8 Fiscal responsibility: The evaluator's allocation and expenditure of resources should reflect sound accountability procedures and otherwise be prudent and ethically responsible so that expenditures are accounted for and appropriate.

Utility Standards

The utility standards are intended to ensure that an evaluation will serve the information needs of intended users.

U1 Stakeholder identification: Persons involved in or affected by the evaluation should be identified so that their needs can be addressed.

U2 Evaluator credibility: The persons conducting the evaluation should be both trustworthy and competent to perform the evaluation so that the evaluation findings achieve maximum credibility and acceptance.

U3 Information scope and selection: Information collected should be broadly selected to address pertinent questions about the program and be responsive to the needs and interests of clients and other specified stakeholders.

U4 Values identification: The perspectives, procedures, and rationale used to interpret the findings should be carefully described so that the bases for value judgments are clear.

U5 Report clarity: Evaluation reports should clearly describe the program being evaluated, including its context and the purposes, procedures, and findings of the evaluation, so that essential information is provided and easily understood.

U6 Report timeliness and dissemination: Significant interim findings and evaluation reports should be disseminated to intended users so that they can be used in a timely fashion.

U7 Evaluation impact: Evaluations should be planned, conducted, and reported in ways that encourage follow-through by stakeholders to increase the likelihood that the evaluation will be used.

Feasibility Standards

The feasibility standards are intended to ensure that an evaluation will be realistic, prudent, diplomatic, and frugal.

F1 Practical procedures: The evaluation procedures should be practical to keep disruption to a minimum while needed information is obtained.

F2 Political viability: The evaluation should be planned and conducted with anticipation of the different positions of various interest groups so that their cooperation may be obtained and so that possible attempts by any of these groups to curtail evaluation operations or to bias or misapply the results can be averted or counteracted.

F3 Cost effectiveness: The evaluation should be efficient and produce information of sufficient value so that the resources expended can be justified.

Accuracy Standards

The accuracy standards are intended to ensure that an evaluation will reveal and convey technically adequate information about the features that determine worth or merit of the program being evaluated.

A1 Program documentation: The program being evaluated should be described and documented clearly and accurately so that the program is clearly identified.

A2 Context analysis: The context in which the program exists should be examined in enough detail that its likely influences on the program can be identified.

A3 Described purposes and procedures: The purposes and procedures of the evaluation should be monitored and described in enough detail that they can be identified and assessed.

A4 Defensible information sources: The sources of information used in a program evaluation should be described in enough detail that the adequacy of the information can be assessed.

A5 Valid information: The information gathering procedures should be chosen or developed and then implemented in a way that ensures the interpretation arrived at is valid for the intended use.

A6 Reliable information: The information gathering procedures should be chosen or developed and then implemented in a way that ensures the information obtained is sufficiently reliable for the intended use.

A7 Systematic information: The information collected, processed, and reported in an evaluation should be systematically reviewed and any errors found should be corrected.

A8 Analysis of quantitative information: Quantitative information in an evaluation should be appropriately and systematically analyzed so that evaluation questions are effectively answered.

A9 Analysis of qualitative information: Qualitative information in an evaluation should be appropriately and systematically analyzed so that evaluation questions are effectively answered.

A10 Justified conclusions: The conclusions reached in an evaluation should be explicitly justified so that stakeholders can assess them.

A11 Impartial reporting: Reporting procedures should guard against distortion caused by personal feelings and biases of any party to the evaluation so that evaluation reports fairly reflect the evaluation findings.

A12 Meta-evaluation: The evaluation itself should be formatively and summatively evaluated against these and other pertinent standards so that its conduct is appropriately guided and stakeholders can closely examine its strengths and weaknesses upon completion.

Additional Resource:

Sanders JR. *The Program Evaluation Standards: How to Assess Evaluations of Educational Programs.* 2d ed. Newbury Park, CA: Sage; 1994.

APPENDIX C:
ADDITIONAL INFORMATION ON THE PURPOSE, SELECTION, AND ROLES OF THE EVALUATION ADVISORY GROUP

Why establish an advisory group?

A fundamental element in the 10-step process is inclusion and engagement of an evaluation advisory group. This advisory group becomes critical in ensuring that the evaluation is participatory in nature.

Given that the purpose of evaluation is to provide useful information for program improvement and decision making, the key challenge is identifying and prioritizing what information and data would be most useful. Everything else flows from this initial determination—methods, measures, focus, analysis, and reporting. An evaluator, acting alone, may miss some important and relevant issues. Key stakeholders that are connected with a program at different levels and in various ways can provide different perspectives on what is important and useful to know. By bringing these perspectives together to inform the evaluation, each person in a collaboration makes a contribution—and each benefits.

An effective method for engaging stakeholders is to create an advisory group to participate in the design and implementation of the evaluation and to help determine what actions are needed, based on the evaluation findings. Increasing evaluation capacity becomes an added benefit of involving an advisory group. As stakeholders come together to discuss different evaluation activities and the results of data collection, they learn how to conduct program evaluations while also learning about each other and the program being evaluated. This experience strengthens personal relationships and increases each participant's ability to think evaluatively and apply what they've learned to future evaluation projects.

How should advisory group members be selected?

Careful consideration should be given to the selection of advisory group members. To ensure that the group is able to function effectively, all advisory group members must agree to commit their time and energy to attending advisory group meetings whenever possible.

The advisory group should include representatives from the following groups:

- Staff who have administrative oversight of the program;
- Staff who are responsible for the daily operations of the program;
- Current or future recipients of program services;
- Stakeholders who are diverse in terms of class, gender, and age;
- Representatives of organizations interested in the outcomes of the evaluation;

- Staff who will be responsible for implementing the evaluation's recommendations and action plan; and
- Staff who have some experience with evaluation.

In selecting advisory group members, it is a good idea to involve people who bring variety in terms of their (1) views of the program, (2) intended uses of the evaluation results, (3) positions within the organization and community, and (4) experience with the program being evaluated. In addition, it is important that at least some of the team members have an understanding of the politics of the organization and the program.

How many people should be on the advisory group?

The number of people on an advisory group will vary depending on the scope of the evaluation and the nature of the program being evaluated. Typically, advisory groups composed of 5 to 10 members are sufficient to create enough synergy and dialogue to keep the process going.

What is the role of the advisory group?

The advisory group's function is to provide advice throughout the evaluation, to help the evaluator think through various program issues, to review drafts of the evaluation plan and data collection instruments, to provide insights into the collected data, and to make recommendations based on the evaluation's findings. The group's role is a reflective one, not one of making final decisions about the evaluation's design, implementation, or final report. In addition, the advisory group provides insights into the social and political context of the program being evaluated.

Members should meet to discuss the background of the program and develop the evaluation's rationale, purpose statement, stakeholders, and key questions to be addressed. This first meeting is critical to getting the evaluation focused in a way that will address the decision-making needs of the stakeholders. This meeting should be scheduled for a minimum of two hours. Although this meeting can take place via a conference call, ideally the advisory group will meet face-to-face at least twice during the evaluation process. In between these meetings, members may be asked to perform additional tasks.

Advisory group members should individually review the draft evaluation plan that is prepared by the evaluation facilitator and the evaluator.

Once the data collection instruments have been developed, the members should individually review the instruments to ensure that the key evaluation questions are addressed and the questions or items are well constructed.

When the evaluator has completed the data collection phase and has aggregated the data, the advisory group should be reconvened for another face-to-face meeting. During this meeting, the evaluator facilitates a discussion of the evaluation's findings and engages the group in a process of analyzing the findings. Typically, this discussion leads to development of a set of recommendations that the evaluator will incorporate into the final report. This meeting may last from two to six hours, depending on the quantity of information collected during the evaluation and the complexity of the evaluation findings.

After the evaluation report has been written, consider establishing a task force that will develop an action plan for implementing the evaluation's recommendations. This task force might be composed of the same people who served on the advisory group or it might be a combination of advisory group members and others who have more contact with the program's daily operations. If original advisory group members are not involved in the task force, it is important they understand why. All group members should always be thanked for their original participation.

APPENDIX D:
PROCESS EVALUATION QUESTIONS AND LOGIC MODEL FROM THE CENTER FOR TOBACCO POLICY RESEARCH

This appendix includes an example of a logic model for a process evaluation provided by the Center for Tobacco Policy Research (CTPR), Saint Louis University School of Public Health (see also **Exhibit D-1** on page 71).

The CTPR evaluated a tobacco prevention and cessation initiative funded by the Missouri Foundation for Health. One of the initiative's strategies focused on an educational campaign to increase awareness among the general population about the dangers of tobacco in order to help gain public support for an increase in the state's tobacco tax. The evaluation also addressed numerous questions about the inputs, activities, and outputs of this initiative. Some of the questions that the evaluation was intended to answer through analysis of inputs, activities, and outputs appear below.

Inputs

- Were the resources for the educational campaign adequate?
- Who were the collaborators for the campaign? How effective were both the existing and new collaborations?

Activities

- What was the level of communication among stakeholders?
- Was there sufficient (or effective) communication among stakeholders?
- How was the campaign developed and implemented?
- Was the education campaign prepared for (and flexible enough) to respond to environmental changes?

Outputs

- What was the reach of the grassroots education activities?
- How many advocacy committees were developed?
- How many volunteers were recruited?
- What was the geographic coverage of the campaign?
- How many people received the education messages?
- What were the responses from various audiences to the education messages?
- Were the messages appropriate for different audiences?

Introduction to Process Evaluation in Tobacco Use Prevention and Control

Exhibit D-1: Strategy 1 Logic Model: Show Me Health—Clearing the Air About Tobacco

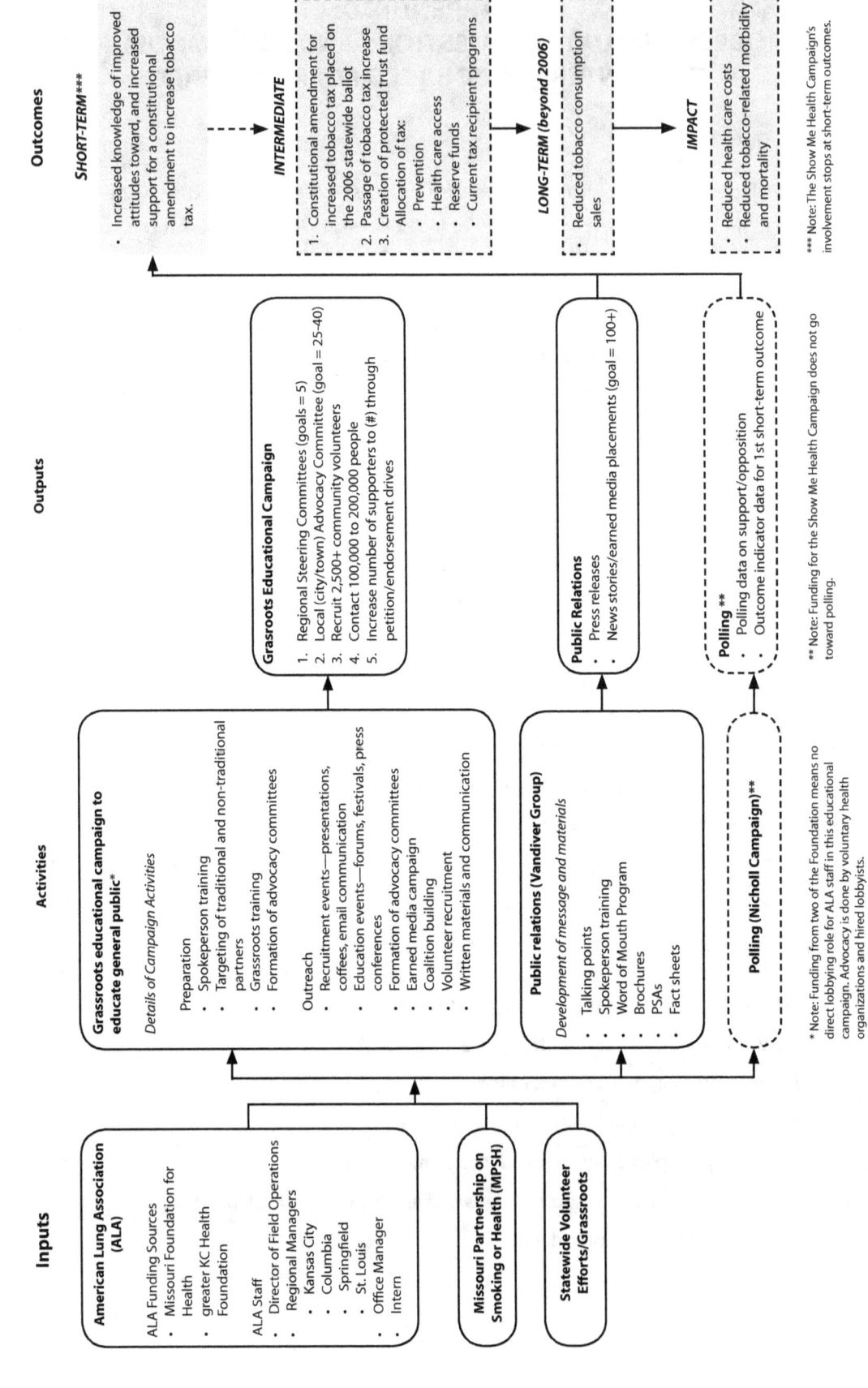

REFERENCES

1. Centers for Disease Control and Prevention. *Best Practices for Comprehensive Tobacco Control Programs.* Atlanta GA: U.S. Department of Health and Human Services; August 1999.

2. MacDonald G, Starr G, Schooley M, Yee SS, Klimowski K, Turner K. *Introduction to Program Evaluation for Comprehensive Tobacco Control Programs.* Atlanta, GA: U.S. Department of Health and Human Services; 2001.

3. Starr G, Rogers T, Schooley M, Porter S, Wiesen E, Jamison N. *Key Outcome Indicators for Evaluating Comprehensive Tobacco Control Programs.* Atlanta, GA: U.S. Department of Health and Human Services; 2005.

4. Centers for Disease Control and Prevention. Framework for program evaluation in public health. *MMWR* 1999b;48(RR11):1–40.

5. Mueller N, Luke D, Herbers S, Montgomery T. The best practices: Use of the guidelines by ten state tobacco control programs.American Journal of Preventive Medicine 2006;31(4).

6. Zaza S, Harris KW, Briss PA, editors. *The Guide to Community Preventive Services: What Works to Promote Health.* Task Force on Community Preventive Services; 2004.

7. California Department of Health Services, Tobacco Control Section. *Communities of Excellence in Tobacco Control* (Modules 1 and 2). Pre-production copy; September 2006.

8. Patton MQ. *Utilization-Focused Evaluation: The New Century Text.* 2nd edition. Newbury Park, CA: Sage; 1986.

9. Steckler A, Linnan L, editors. *Process Evaluation for Public Health Interventions and Research.* San Francisco, CA: Jossey-Bass; 2002.

10. Patton MQ. The CEFP as a model for integrating evaluation within organizations. Cancer Practice 2001;9(1): S11-S16.

11. Compton D, Baizerman M, editors. Managing Program Evaluation: Towards Explicating a Professional Orientation and Practice. *New Directions for Evaluation* (forthcoming).

12. Compton DW, Baizerman M, Preskill H, Rieker P, Miner K. Developing evaluation capacity while improving evaluation training in public health: The American Cancer Society's Collaborative Evaluation Fellows Project. *Evaluation and Program Planning* 2001;24 (1):33–40.

13. Torres R, Preskill H, Piontek M. *Evaluation Strategies for Communicating and Learning: Enhancing Learning in Organizations.* Thousand Oaks, CA: Sage Publications, Inc.; 1996.

14. Sanders JR. Joint Committee on Standards for Educational Evaluation. *The Program Evaluation Standards: How to Assess Educational Programs.* 2nd Edition. Thousand Oaks, CA: Sage Publications, Inc.; 1994.

15. Patton MQ. *Qualitative Evaluation and Research Methods.* 2nd ed. Thousand Oaks, CA: Sage Publications, Inc.; 1990.

16. Weiss CH. On theory-based evaluation: Winning friends and influencing people. *The Evaluation Exchange* 2004;IX(4):1-5.

17. Mattessich P. *The Manager's Guide to Program Evaluation: Planning, Contracting, and Managing for Useful Results.* Saint Paul, MN: Amherst H. Wilder Foundation; 2003.

18. NVivo 7. QSR International, Inc.

19. Atlas.ti. Scientific Software Development GmbH.

20. Greene JC. Stakeholder participation in utilization of evaluation. *Evaluation Review* 1988;12:2.

21. Compton DW, Baizerman M, Stockdill SH, editors. The art, craft, and science of evaluation capacity building: *New Directions for Evaluation* 2002;93.

www.ingramcontent.com/pod-product-compliance
Lightning Source LLC
Chambersburg PA
CBHW081738170526
45167CB00009B/3862